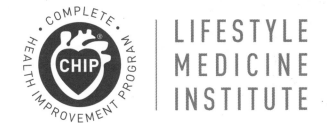

LIFESTYLE
MEDICINE
INSTITUTE

Beginning Your CHIP Journey

I, ...

began my CHIP journey on .... at ....

I began my CHIP journey because

....

....

By the end of the first three months of my CHIP journey I would like to be able to

....

....

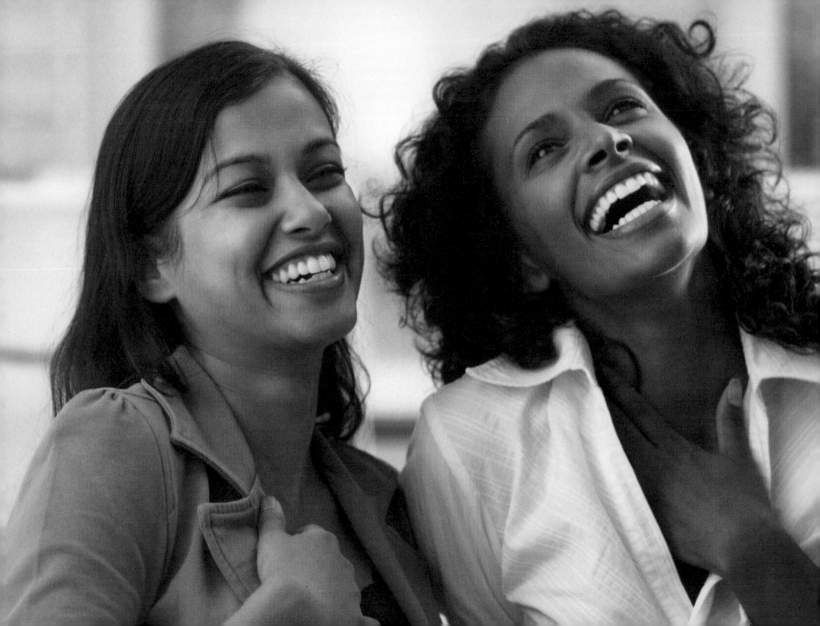

Welcome

It has been a great joy for me to be part of the team responsible for the development of the Complete Health Improvement Program (CHIP). CHIP represents the creative energy of many talented individuals, including medical doctors, nutritionists, exercise physiologists, psychologists, health promoters and educators. But while these contributors have different areas of expertise, they have a common interest—helping you to live more.

CHIP has been developed with you in mind. Its purpose is to guide you on a journey of transformation by providing you with a vision of the healthy life you deserve. CHIP offers the best and most up-to-date information on how to achieve it, the necessary resources and support to keep you motivated along the way, and a well thought through action plan to get you there. Indeed, CHIP offers you the best chance of success!

But there is something else unique about CHIP. It is called the Complete Health Improvement Program for good reason as it addresses all aspects of health including nutrition, physical activity, substance use, stress, self-worth and even happiness. After all, what's the point of being healthy if you're miserable?

In CHIP you will be given all the pieces of the puzzle required to truly flourish.

The CHIP team would love to be there alongside you as you progress through the program, and it is through this workbook that we get to. I encourage you to really engage with this workbook in the weeks to come. Give it your best effort. CHIP works—and it can work for you. You deserve it, too!

Today is the first day of the rest of your life and it offers a new beginning. I truly hope you take the CHIP challenge and choose to live your best life. Let CHIP help you live more!

Darren Morton

Darren Morton, PhD
Lifestyle Education Research Group
Avondale College of Higher Education

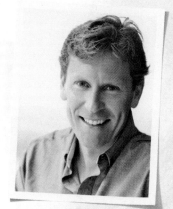

Your CHIP Presenters

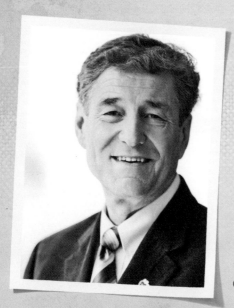

Dr Hans Diehl

Hans Diehl is the founder of the Lifestyle Medicine Institute in Loma Linda, California, where he is clinical professor of Preventive Medicine at the School of Medicine of Loma Linda University. The clinical results of his pioneering efforts as an epidemiologically trained lifestyle interventionist with his CHIP program have been published in more than 20 peer-reviewed medical journals. The New York Academy of Medicine listed this program among the top three proven community-based prevention programs in the United States. More than 50,000 graduates have learned how simple lifestyle changes can facilitate the prevention and even the reversal of many of our common modern killer diseases.

Hans holds a Doctorate in Health Science and a Masters in Public Health Nutrition from Loma Linda University. He had a fellowship as a post-doctoral scholar at the University of California at Los Angeles and a two-year research fellowship in cardiovascular epidemiology sponsored by the National Institutes of Health.

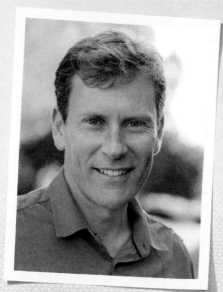

Dr Darren Morton

Darren Morton is a senior lecturer in the Faculty of Education and Science at Avondale College of Higher Education in Cooranbong, New South Wales, Australia, where he has been based since 1994.

Darren has a PhD in Human Physiology and his present research passion is the emerging field of Lifestyle Medicine. He has numerous publications and has delivered hundreds of presentations on lifestyle-related topics, nationally and internationally.

Darren enjoys family time, hang-gliding and triathlon, and is passionate about empowering others to live more.

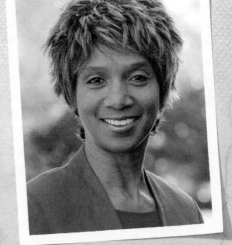

Dr Andrea Avery

Andrea Avery is an Internal Medicine physician with more than 25 years of clinical experience. She has an extensive background in both private practice and academic medicine. She has authored and co-authored several journal articles, as well as conducted clinical pharmacologic research. She has served on the faculties of Wright State University, Thomas Jefferson University, and most recently, as Professor of Medicine at University of California, Irvine. Her interests include clinical teaching, preventive care and women's health, as well as exercise and fitness.

How to get the most out of your CHIP experience

This workbook forms the backbone of your CHIP experience and it will serve as a companion and guide as you journey through the program. It is here that the rubber meets the road—you get to put theory into practice and reflect on what you have learned from session to session.

To maximize your experience, it is imperative that you engage with this workbook, and as you do you will find recurring themes in each session:

 DISCOVER

Focuses on the key points of each session and, in particular, what is new to you.

 EXPERIENCE

Issues a challenge that involves putting into practice what you have learned.

 EXPLORE

Reflects on how well you went with the challenge. What worked and what didn't? What would you do differently next time? What would you do the same?

 SHARE

Invites you to share your experience with your CHIP friends so you can learn from and support each other. You will also be challenged to be an agent of positive change within your family and among your wider circle of influence, by sharing in practical ways your journey toward better health.

Don't forget that your CHIP facilitator is there to guide your CHIP journey, so be sure to make use of their support!

Live*more*

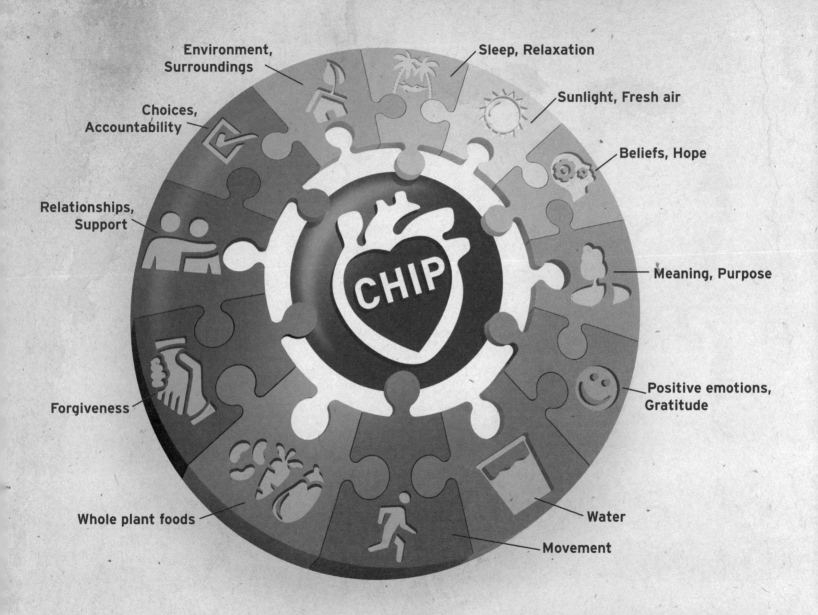

Environment, Surroundings

Sleep, Relaxation

Choices, Accountability

Sunlight, Fresh air

Beliefs, Hope

Relationships, Support

CHIP

Meaning, Purpose

Forgiveness

Positive emotions, Gratitude

Whole plant foods

Water

Movement

Whole Person Health

Part of the CHIP philosophy is that true health–whole person health–is like a jigsaw puzzle, with a number of different pieces that come together to create a whole. Throughout CHIP, you will be guided on how to put this jigsaw together in the context of your own health, helping you to live a truly happy, healthy life. As individuals, we're all at different stages of finishing this puzzle and many of us already have some of these pieces in place. Even if this is the case, we'd encourage you to really think about the whole of health during your CHIP journey, taking full advantage of all of the tools presented in this program. Looking deeper at the pieces we already have in place can often help us realize how other pieces fit next to them, bringing life to the whole picture.

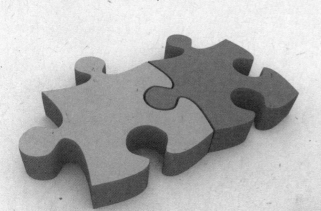

Check out <www.vimeo.com/chiphealth> for some great tips on grocery shopping for health.

Session One

The Rise and Rise of Chronic Disease

✿ DISCOVER

› What three things have you learned?

....

....

....

....

....

....

....

› Why are you doing CHIP?

....

....

....

....

....

....

....

"Health is not everything, but without it, everything is nothing!"

> What might your future be like if you don't make changes to your lifestyle?

....

....

....

....

....

> If you do make positive lifestyle changes, how will it affect your life and future?

....

....

....

....

....

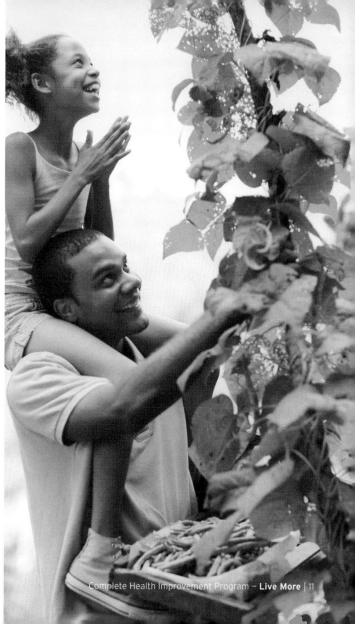

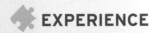 **EXPERIENCE**

Start *JumpStart* within the next 48 hours

What is the 5-Day *JumpStart* Challenge?

The 5-Day *JumpStart* Challenge is designed to prepare you physically and mentally to experience the benefits of improved health.

This 5-Day *JumpStart* Challenge is an integral part of the Complete Health Improvement Program (CHIP) and is recommended to everyone needing a lifestyle makeover. Even though considerable testing has shown this plan to be a sensible, prudent and safe approach, people with significant health problems, such as diabetes or other chronic diseases should check with their doctors before beginning. Except for this 5-Day *JumpStart* Challenge, CHIP does not provide specific menus or meal plans. The emphasis is on learning to eat and live for optimal health and wellbeing using the *Optimal Diet* principles for life!

For people who are stressed, overweight, out of control or suffering from circulatory diseases, this five-day challenge is an excellent starting point. After experiencing the exhilaration and wellbeing resulting from one week of simple eating and good health habits, motivation becomes high and jump starts the *Optimal Diet* principles of CHIP toward a healthier lifestyle.

Dr Diehl's Reality Checks

1. **On the move!** With the *JumpStart* diet, you may experience differences in bowel movements. This is good and the way it should be!

2. **Noting the bloating.** After about a week you may notice an increase in gas or wind. Rest assured, it's only temporary!

3. **Resist and persist.** During this time you may experience headaches, often due to caffeine withdrawal. Stick with it, it will pass!

4. **Lifting the fog.** You may feel mentally sharper, enjoy a better memory and feel better prepared for life's challenges.

5. **Rise and shine.** Getting into the pattern of "early to bed, early to rise" may take some time, but it's worth it!

Benefits of the 5-Day *JumpStart* Challenge

1. **Improves intestinal tract function.** The high fiber content of the food absorbs water in the intestinal tract, turning insoluble fiber into a gel-like substance that resembles a soft, spongy mass. Fiber stimulates intestinal activity and sweeps along intestinal contents more efficiently and effectively.

2. **Decreases fluid retention.** It removes excess water, salt and other toxins from the body via kidneys and intestinal tract.

3. **Helps break food addictions.**

4. **Improves appetite and intensifies taste perception.** It will help you discover and enjoy new flavors in simple foods.

5. **Renews energy and improves mental acuity.** Beginning with Days 3 and 4, energy levels and a sense of wellbeing substantially increase.

6. **Conquers fear.** Since many people in weight-loss programs fear food deprivation and hunger, the 5-Day *JumpStart* Challenge will help handle these feelings and overcome these fears.

7. **Eliminates body odors.** Body odors and bad breath will diminish over time.

8. **Provides a taste of success.** Experience the joy that comes from experimenting with new foods and health-promoting activities.

9. **Reduces food budget.** This new, simpler way of eating can reduce your weekly food costs.

10. **JumpStarts you into a healthier lifestyle!** It begins the establishment of a new way of life and puts you back in control!

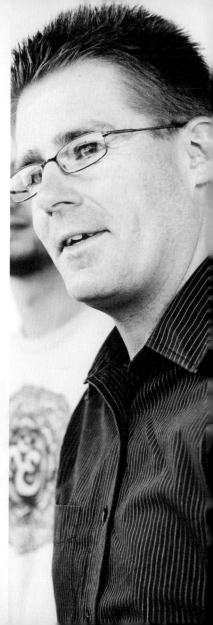

Notes for People with Diabetes

If you have diabetes, start the *JumpStart* Challenge at Day 3 (skip Days 1 and 2).

If on insulin or other medications for diabetes, stay in regular or daily contact with your doctor or diabetes nurse educator to monitor your blood-sugar levels and medication requirements. (For example, insulin dosage often has to be reduced by 2–3 units a day.)

High-fiber, unrefined carbohydrates can be used:

› Due to their high-fiber content, breakfast should focus on whole grain cereals, such as rolled oats or rolled barley. Use as close to the whole grain kernel as possible.

› Eat no more than five slices of bread per day and choose whole grain.

Nuts can be used:

› ¼ cup nuts per day, such as almonds or walnuts, and 1-2 tablespoons of ground flaxseed at breakfast will help satiety and aid in blood-sugar control.

Fruits should be restricted to three servings per day and ideally be eaten with high-fiber dishes:

› Include fresh fruit, such as apples, pears, peaches, apricots and berries.

› Dried fruits and fruit juices should be limited because of their concentrated sugar content.

› Where possible, eat fruit and vegetables with the skin for a higher fiber intake.

Make good use of legumes:

› Use cooked legumes (beans and lentils) with main meals (including breakfast). The high fiber will help lower blood-sugar levels.

NOTES FOR PEOPLE WITH HIGH BLOOD PRESSURE

If you are on medication for high blood pressure, talk with your doctor about monitoring and adjusting your medications as needed.

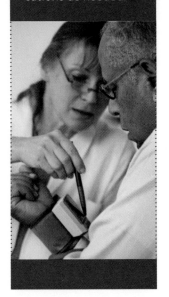

Withdrawal Symptoms

Most people experience some degree of withdrawal for two to five days as a result of food and/or caffeine or nicotine addictions. Transient symptoms may include headache, nausea, fatigue, depression, generalized aching, excessive gas and diarrhea. Headaches will be worse if addicted to caffeine and nicotine.

NOTE: Hang in there for this difficult period. It won't last forever! You'll feel much better once you have made the transition!

Tips on Handling Withdrawal Symptoms

1. **Drink two glasses of water first thing in the morning.** Add a twist of lemon for taste.

2. **Walk briskly outdoors for 15 minutes or more.**

3. **Eat a good breakfast.**

4. **For headaches,** soak feet and legs in hot water for 10-15 minutes. Rinse off with cold water. Rinse a wash cloth in iced water and apply to forehead.

5. **Diarrhea usually settles down in a few days.** If troublesome, take 2-3 charcoal tablets or capsules between meals until the situation normalizes. Ensure fluid intake is increased.

Daily Routine Tips

1. **Just after you wake up in the morning, drink a couple of glasses of water.** Take some time to reflect on the day, think about your goals and choose to be the best you can be for the day.

2. **Take a warm shower or bath before breakfast.**

3. **Ideally eat three meals a day, spaced at least four hours apart.** Make your evening meal the smallest.

4. **Aim to eat your evening meal at least three hours before going to bed.**

5. **At meal time, eat until you feel comfortable and satisfied.**

6. **Avoid eating in front of the TV and, if possible, eat most meals with family or friends.**

7. **Drink at least eight glasses of water or herbal teas each day.** Drink first thing in the morning and between meals.

8. **Develop regularity.** Go to bed, get up, exercise and have your meals at about the same time each day.

9. **Exercise actively for 30-60 minutes each day.** Select an exercise appropriate for your age and condition. Start slowly, increasing time and distance gradually as tolerated.

10. **Allow adequate time for rest.** Aim for eight hours sleep a night and "early to bed, early to rise".

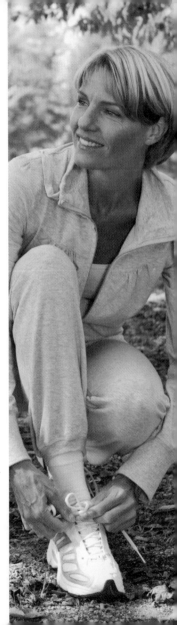

5-Day JumpStart Challenge

Days 1 and 2
Eat fruit and whole grains.

Start here if you have diabetes.

Days 3 to 5
Eat fruit and whole grains plus vegetables and legumes.

After completing Day 5 of the *JumpStart* Challenge, continue with the *Optimal Diet* principles listed on page 6 of *Eat More*.

Throughout all 5 days

› Omit refined sugars, honey, molasses and other concentrated sweeteners.

› Gradually decrease caffeinated drinks.

› Quit all alcohol, fruit juices and soda/soft drinks.

› Omit processed fats and oils, including margarine, butter, mayonnaise, oily dressings and vegetable oils.

› Avoid processed foods and fast foods.

› Leave out animal foods, such as fish, red and white meat.

› Leave out dairy products and eggs. Instead of milk, use nondairy options that are fortified with calcium and B12, such as soy milk or rice milk. If fortified options are not available, or you choose to make your own milk, be sure to include calcium and vitamin B12 supplements in your diet.

› Avoid salt. Season with onion, garlic, ginger, herbs and spices, such as cinnamon, cilantro/coriander or cumin.

› Avoid eating between meals. When hungry, settle for a glass of water or herbal tea. In emergencies, rely on a piece of fresh fruit.

NOTE: The more thoroughly and conscientiously you implement these principles, the more impressive and convincing will be your benefits.

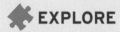 **EXPLORE**

Read *Learn More*, Chapter One

> From your experiences and observations, what do you consider the most important factors in the dramatic increase in chronic diseases in today's society?

....

....

....

....

> In what ways is it true to say that "Modernization itself can be seen as a major contributor to a range of chronic diseases" (*Learn More*, page 7)?

....

....

....

....

....

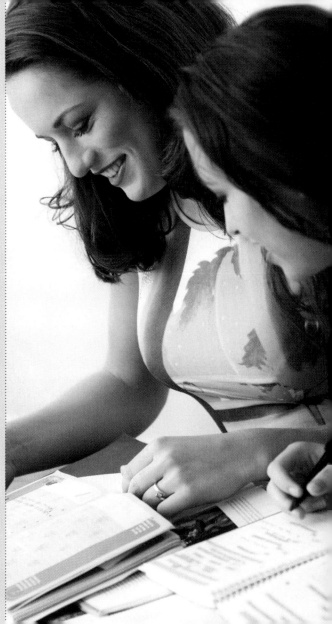

> What positive steps toward healthy lifestyle do you see in your community?

....

....

....

....

> What are some of the ways in which chronic diseases cost us, our families, our communities and our society?

....

....

....

....

> Think about your recent visits to your family doctor or other medical practitioner. With your growing knowledge of "lifestyle medicine," what lifestyle factors or choices may have contributed to your medical need or illness?

....

....

....

> What does it mean to you to be healthy?

....

....

....

SHARE

Share with your CHIP group why you are doing CHIP.

Until the next session, keep notes of your weekly changes on page 152, recording what you change, and what has worked well—or not so well—for you in making these changes.

Session Two

Lifestyle is the Best Medicine

⚙ DISCOVER

› What three things have you learned?

....

....

....

....

....

....

....

....

› Refer to your response in the last session to "What might your future be like if you don't make changes to your lifestyle?" How does it make you feel?

....

....

....

....

....

....

....

....

"As I see it, every day you do one of two things: build health or produce disease in yourself."

[Adelle Davis]

› Refer to your response in the last session to "If you do make positive lifestyle changes, how will it affect your life and future?" How does it make you feel?

....

....

....

....

....

....

....

....

› How does it make you feel to know that by doing CHIP you are making a positive impact on your health?

....

....

....

....

....

....

....

....

"Lifestyle disease is a food-borne illness."

[Dr C Esselstyn]

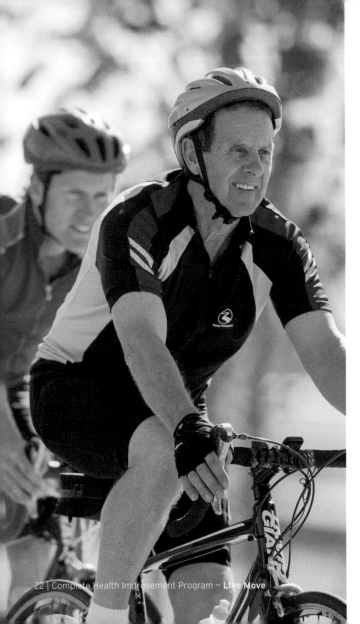

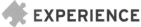 **EXPERIENCE**

Get moving

One of the recurring factors in lifestyle medicine, whether reducing disease risks or reversing existing conditions, is physical activity. For many of us, our modern lifestyles can easily become sedentary lifestyles—we sit in the car or on public transport, we sit at our desks at work, we sit in front of the TV or computer screens in our homes. We need to get moving.

In your CHIP kit, you will have received a pedometer, which offers one way of tracking the number of steps you take in your daily activities. Alternatively, you can keep a record of the number of minutes of intentional exercise or activity you include in your day. Use the activity record chart in the back of this workbook (see page 148) to monitor your activity achievements. The aim is at least 10,000 steps or 40 minutes of moderate or vigorous intensity activity per day.

If you have not been regularly active, do not expect to achieve these goals in the first week. Begin by incorporating more activity than usual into your daily routines. Keep a track of this day by day—as well as your weekly totals—and plan to increase these measures of physical activity during the coming weeks.

Step it out

A pedometer is an easy but effective way to monitor whether you are moving enough throughout the course of the day. For best results, clip your pedometer to your hip above your right knee, although on your shoe can work well, too. Obviously, if you spend much of your time sitting, you will not record as many steps as if you get mobile.

The commonly cited goal is to achieve 10,000 steps per day. The number of daily steps commonly recommended for children is 13,000 steps for boys and 11,000 steps for girls.[1] Older adults or those with chronic diseases such as heart disease might need to set themselves a slightly lower target.

While pedometers have some limitations—they don't measure the *type* of steps you take or count any of the steps you take if you forget to wear them—they can be motivational. Simply wearing a pedometer commonly results in individuals taking an extra 2000 steps per day, which in one study of low-activity individuals resulted in a reduction of about 1 inch (2.5 centimeters) in waist circumference.[2]

Wearing a pedometer motivates you to seek more movement opportunities and helps reinforce in a measureable way the difference that opting for "incidental activities"—like taking the stairs or walking down the hall to speak to a colleague instead of sending an email—can make to your total step count for the day.

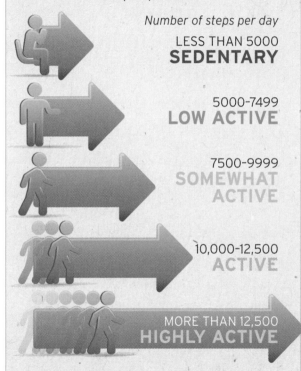

Activity level

Classification of activity level according to daily steps achieved[3]

Number of steps per day

LESS THAN 5000
SEDENTARY

5000-7499
LOW ACTIVE

7500-9999
SOMEWHAT ACTIVE

10,000-12,500
ACTIVE

MORE THAN 12,500
HIGHLY ACTIVE

1 Vincent, S, R P Pangrazi, et al (2003), "Activity Levels and body mass index of children in the United States, Sweden and Australia," *Medicine and Science in Sport and Exercise,* Vol 35 No 8, pages 1367-73.

2 Dwyer, T, et al (2007), "The inverse relationship between number of steps per day and obesity in a population-based sample—the AusDiab study," *International Journal of Obesity,* Vol 31, pages 797-804.

3 Tudor-Locke, C, et al (2008) "Revisiting 'how many steps are enough?'" *Medicine and Science in Sports and Exercise,* Vol 40, No 7 Supplement, pages S537-43.

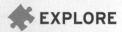 **EXPLORE**

Read *Learn More*, Chapter Two

> Which of the lifestyle research or reversal studies introduced in this
> project most caught your attention? Why?

....

....

....

....

....

....

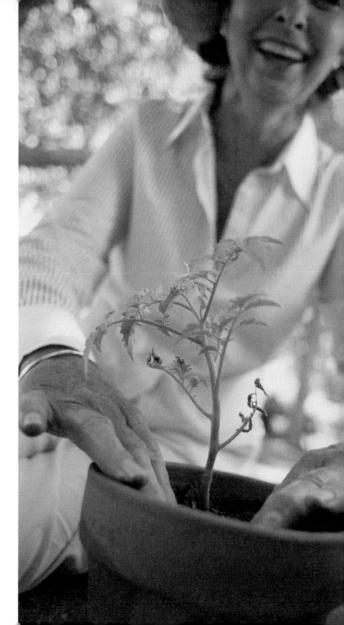

› Is it encouraging to hear others' lives changed through the Complete Health Improvement Program (CHIP) and other lifestyle interventions for disease reversal? Why?

....

....

....

....

....

....

› True or false? Equipped with the information in this program, you can cancel your next appointment with your regular doctor. Explain your answer.

....

....

....

....

....

Until the next session, keep notes of your weekly changes on page 152, recording what you change, and what has worked well—or not so well—for you in making these changes.

SHARE

Explain "Lifestyle medicine" to a friend who is unfamiliar with the term.

Session Three

The Common Denominator of Chronic Disease

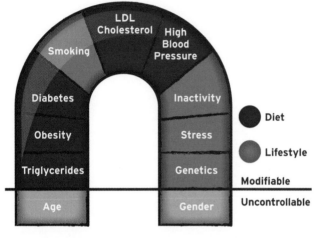

Diet

Lifestyle

Modifiable

Uncontrollable

LDL Cholesterol · High Blood Pressure · Smoking · Diabetes · Inactivity · Obesity · Stress · Triglycerides · Genetics · Age · Gender

🧩 DISCOVER

› What three things have you learned about the causes of chronic disease?

....

....

....

....

....

....

› With the understanding you have gained in this session, which of the risk factors of chronic lifestyle disease concern you most?

....

....

....

....

> "Oxidative stress," "antioxidants" and "free radicals" are terms we often hear in advertising for health products and foods. How would you explain each of these in a simple way?

Oxidative stress

....

....

Antioxidants

....

....

Free radicals

....

....

Dr Darren Morton undergoes an experiment in oxidative stress at <www.vimeo.com/chiphealth>.

> Is the idea of a whole range of chronic diseases caused by one thing—lifestyle—troubling or helpful? Why?

....

....

....

....

....

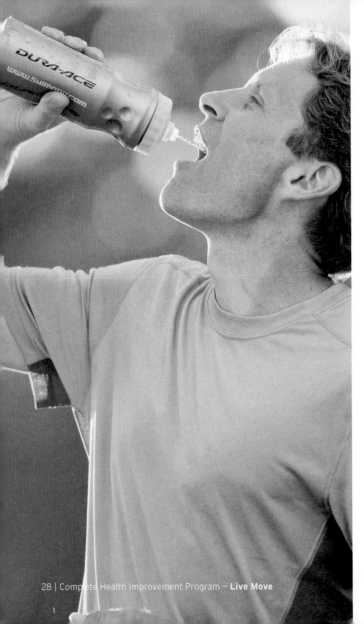

 EXPERIENCE

Drink 8 glasses of water today

For all of us, water is necessary for life—it's that simple. Water is crucial in a range of metabolic processes. It is found in all the cells in our body and is an important ingredient to keep our body functioning at its best. Fluid passing through the body is also an important way waste products are removed from the body.

If we are not drinking enough water, we can become lethargic and experience symptoms of mild dehydration, such as headaches. Dehydration—when our water levels are running low—results in a decrease in blood volume, which can lead to low blood pressure, dizziness and even fainting. In extreme cases, it can even lead to delirium, unconsciousness and death.

Exact requirements for water differ from person to person but what remains common is that we need plenty of water each day. While some of this water is provided by the foods we eat, getting eight glasses of water a day is the best way to make up the difference.

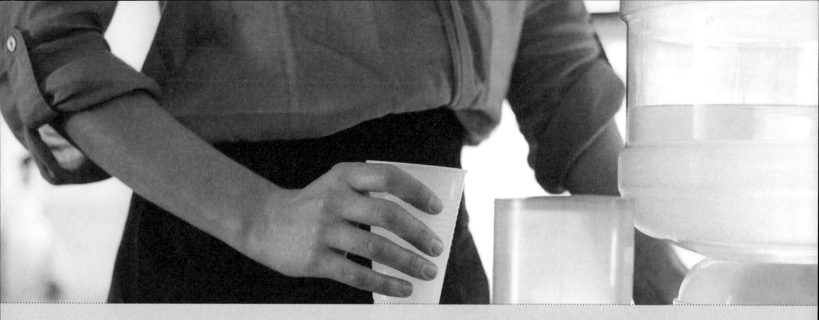

TIPS FOR DRINKING MORE WATER

1 **Keep a water bottle with you during the day,** perhaps at your desk, in the car or wherever it will be within easy reach. This helps you keep track of how much you've drunk through the day and is a visual reminder.

2 **Keep your water cold.** Many people find the taste and refreshing nature of cold water more appealing than room-temperature water.

3 **Spice it up.** Some people find the taste of water boring, so try adding a slice of lemon or lime to your water to bring it to life without filling it with calories.

4 **Hourly reminder.** Set a reminder on your phone or computer at work to go off every hour to remind you to drink a glass of water.

5 **Try drinking a glass of water before each meal.** Meal times work as a good reminder and drinking water helps fill you up, while containing no calories.

6 **Start the day hydrated.** Drink two glasses of water every morning after waking up.

7 **After going to the bathroom, drink a glass of water.**

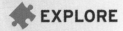 **EXPLORE**

Read *Learn More,* Chapter Three

> What lifestyle choices are you practising that would combat inflammation, lowering your risk of chronic disease?

....

....

....

....

> How is this explanation of heart disease different to what you previously understood?

....

....

....

....

> Why is it important to understand how our mind and body work together?

....

....

....

....

> What questions are raised in your mind by the information in this chapter?

....

....

....

....

› Try writing your own "lifestyle medicine prescription." Be as specific as possible with the information you have—and be prepared to fine-tune this as you continue on your journey to a healthier lifestyle.

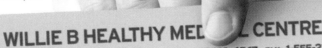

Rx

WILLIE B HEALTHY MEDICAL CENTRE
123 Hy Gene Court, Chipville ID 90382   PHONE: 1-555-123-4567   FAX: 1-555-234-5678

Name .... Date ....

Positive Lifestyle Change ....

....

....

Frequency..

Amount ....

By signing this prescription I agree to commit to giving full effort to my lifestyle change

Signature ....

Until the next session, keep notes of your weekly changes on page 153, recording what you change, and what has worked well—or not so well—for you in making these changes.

SHARE

Share your "lifestyle prescription" with a family member or someone in your CHIP group.

Find Dr Darren Morton's participant challenge at <www.vimeo.com/chiphealth>.

The Optimal Lifestyle

✂ DISCOVER

› What three things have you learned about the Optimal Lifestyle?

› Thinking about the food you ate when you were a child, is your diet healthier then or now? What are the three most significant changes?

> *"To insure good health: eat lightly, breathe deeply, live moderately, cultivate cheerfulness, and maintain an interest in life."*
>
> [William Londen]

> On a scale of 1 (least important) to 10 (most important), rate the importance of each of the following to your current food choices:

Convenience   1 2 3 4 5 6 7 8 9 10

Price   1 2 3 4 5 6 7 8 9 10

Taste   1 2 3 4 5 6 7 8 9 10

Culture or habits   1 2 3 4 5 6 7 8 9 10

Health   1 2 3 4 5 6 7 8 9 10

Environmental impact   1 2 3 4 5 6 7 8 9 10

> Why are diet and activity equally important in achieving the optimal lifestyle?

....

....

....

....

....

> What are the three most important ways exercise can help you feel better about yourself?

....

....

....

....

....

....

> What steps toward health have you been motivated to take today?

....

....

....

....

Poor Health Outcomes

←

POOR HEALTH CHOICES

 EXPERIENCE

> **Choose where you want to be on the health spectrum**

The spectrum is all about choice. It isn't a matter of all or nothing, but where you choose to be dictates the level of benefit you'll receive. Moving across the spectrum is a journey, but unlike a long walk, this journey gets easier with every step you take. As you learn the principles of CHIP and start working these into your day-to-day life, you will find that you'll start identifying more and more ways to continue your journey that are tailored perfectly for you.

> If you've managed to start drinking more water, you've already taken a positive step along the spectrum!

> Remember, where you choose to be now doesn't have to be where you stay. Some people find that a gradual progression along the spectrum toward healthier choices is more sustainable than one big change.

> Look for quick wins. Think about the meals you normally enjoy and look for easy ways to make them better choices. Maybe you could make that stir-fry you love with brown rice instead of white, or you might be able to use lentils in your favourite pasta dish instead of mince meat. Healthy eating doesn't have to mean changing everything you eat.

Optimal Health Outcomes

POSITIVE HEALTH CHOICES

> Be honest about what you are willing to do. It's easy to say we are going to change our diets all in one go, then find it too hard and revert to old habits, feeling dejected.

> Take things one step at a time. Some people find that choosing one or two changes or improvements each week leads to greater long-term success.

> Be prepared to experiment with healthy choices. Choose one lifestyle habit and pursue it for a few weeks, taking note of the benefits and other changes you notice in your life, your health and how you feel.

INCLUDING:

FRUITS

VEGETABLES

LEGUMES

WHOLE GRAINS

WATER

PHYSICAL ACTIVITY

REST

NUTS*

*include a small handful or only ¼ cup per day

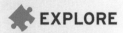 **EXPLORE**

Read *Learn More*, Chapter Ten

> What are the three things that make you less active today than at some previous stage in your life?

....

....

....

....

> How much "screen time" do you spend in an average day or week?

....

....

....

....

....

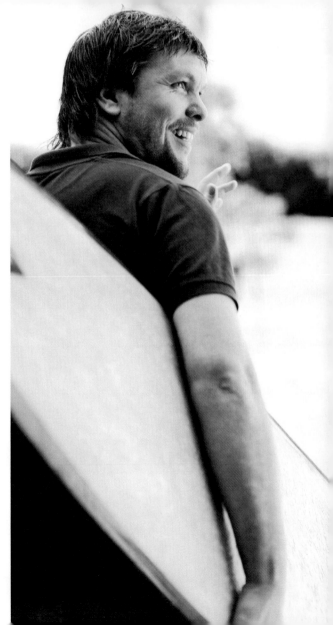

> What is one thing you could do to reduce this inactive time and replace it with activity?

....

....

....

> What is the difference between exercise and activity? Think of Dan Buettner's description of "moving naturally."

....

....

....

....

> In what important way is it true to say that "exercise is medicine"?

....

....

....

> What are the advantages of exercise over other medicines?

....

....

....

SHARE
Invite someone to join you for a walk.

Until the next session, keep notes of your weekly changes on page 153, recording what you change, and what has worked well—or not so well—for you in making these changes.

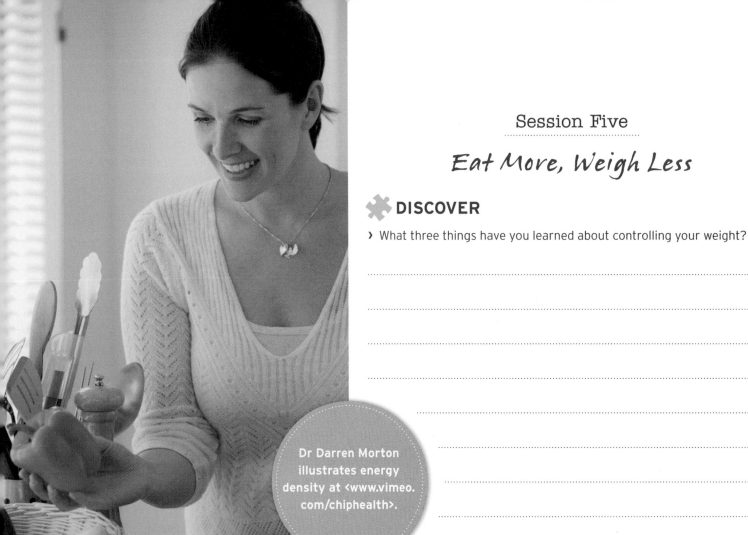

Session Five

Eat More, Weigh Less

DISCOVER

› What three things have you learned about controlling your weight?

....

....

....

....

....

....

....

Dr Darren Morton illustrates energy density at <www.vimeo.com/chiphealth>.

> Why does "dieting"—as commonly understood—often not help with sustainable weight loss?

....

....

....

....

....

> In what ways does the CHIP optimal diet differ from common diets?

....

....

....

....

> What are your dominant emotions and feelings regarding your current weight?

....

....

....

....

....

> What are three triggers, feelings, events or occasions that sometimes cause you to make poor food choices?

....

....

....

....

....

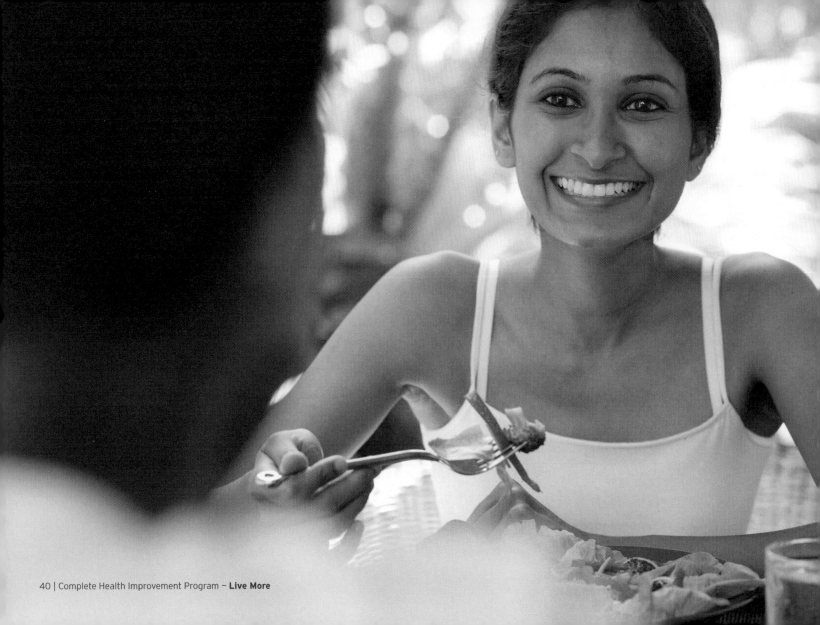

Body Mass Index

While it has some limitations, Body Mass Index (BMI) can be a useful tool for assessing where we fall in the healthy weight range:

How to calculate Body Mass Index

$$\textbf{BMI}_{\text{Imperial}} = \frac{\text{Weight (pounds)}}{\text{Height}^2 \text{ (inches)}} \times \textbf{703} = \underline{\hspace{3cm}}$$

OR

$$\textbf{BMI}_{\text{Metric}} = \frac{\text{Weight (kg)}}{\text{Height}^2 \text{ (m)}} = \underline{\hspace{3cm}}$$

Need to convert pounds to kilograms or inches to centimeters? Check out our quick conversion guide on the inside of your *Live More* back cover.

BMI	Range of weight
Under 18.5	Underweight
18.5 to 24.9	Normal or healthy weight
25.0 to 29.9	Overweight
Over 30.0	Obese

EXPERIENCE

Pantry purge

Removing temptation is key to keeping on track. It's too easy to grab bad choices from the cupboard during or after a busy day and the best way to stop this is to make sure there are no bad choices to grab! Purging your pantry—and refrigerator—gives you a fresh start and a chance to stock your cupboard with healthy staples to build healthy meals from.

> Be ruthless. It can feel wrong to throw away food—many of us grow up being taught not to waste—but some food is better thrown out than eaten. And remember, you won't be doing this every week.

> Make a list of new staple foods to buy. Restocking your pantry with healthy food makes it much easier to create a healthy meal in a hurry. Start investigating recipes you might like, so you can stock your pantry with the kinds of basic ingredients they use.

> Stock up on storage. See *Eat More* (pages 9-11) for a "Kitchen Makeover" shopping list. Grains and dried legumes can be great foods to get savings on in bulk, but they need to be stored in airtight containers once opened. Keeping a stock of these in the pantry helps ensure you won't be caught short when inspiration strikes.

> Keep a notepad next to the pantry, so next time you're cooking and use up the last of one of your staple foods, write it down on the list. This gets rid of some of the stress when it comes to shopping day. Just tear off the top page, rather than having to rummage through the cupboard trying to remember what you've run out of.

It can feel wrong to throw away food—many of us grow up being taught not to waste—but some food is better thrown out than eaten.

Energy density and satiety

Satiety—our feeling of fullness—is strongly influenced by the quantity or volume of food we eat. This is why whole plant foods can help us to eat more and weigh less. Their calories come with bulk, helping us eat more and feel fuller on the same amount of calories compared to energy-dense foods.

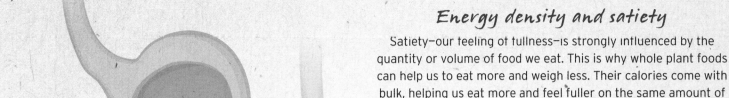

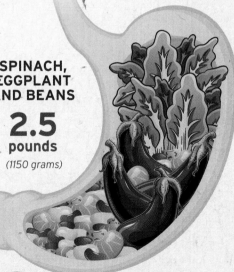

OLIVE OIL

1.6
ounces

(45 grams)

**ROASTED
CHICKEN
DRUMSTICKS
WITH SKIN**

7.6
ounces

(215 grams)

**SPINACH,
EGGPLANT
AND BEANS**

2.5
pounds

(1150 grams)

Each
stomach contains
400
calories
(1672 kJ)

USDA National Nutrient Database for Standard Reference,
<http://www.ars.usda.gov/main/site_main.htm?modecode=12-35-45-00>.

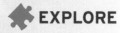 **EXPLORE**

Read *Learn More*, Chapter Four

› How would you convince a friend that they can eat more and weigh less?

....

....

....

....

....

› How are measures such as Body Mass Index or other tables of measures of ideal body weight helpful? What are some of their limitations?

....

....

....

....

SHARE

Explain to a friend or family member the concept of eating more and weighing less (energy density).

› Other than modifying your diet, what other steps might you be able to take to adjust your energy balance—energy in versus energy out?

....

....

....

....

› Explain the term "energy density" and what it should mean for our food choices:

....

....

....

› At what times of the day do you find yourself feeling hungry? Can your day or meals be adapted or rearranged to avoid being hungry when you are more likely to eat less healthy snack foods?

....

....

....

› What have you discovered about your current diet in the process of conducting your "pantry purge"?

....

....

....

....

Until the next session, keep notes of your weekly changes on page 153, recording what you change, and what has worked well—or not so well—for you in making these changes.

Session Six

Fiber, Your New Best Friend

✳ DISCOVER

› What three things have you learned about the importance of fiber in the diet?

....

....

....

....

....

....

....

....

› Was it a surprise to learn that there is no fiber in animal-based foods? Why or why not?

....

....

....

....

....

....

....

....

If there were ever a nutritional version of a best friend, it would be fiber.

> What is the significance of drinking adequate water (at least eight glasses per day) for bowel health?

....

....

....

....

> Why is the amount of time food takes to pass through us significant?

....

....

....

....

> How can you manage the potential "gas problem" talked about in this session?

....

....

....

....

> What are three ways you can achieve the goal of eating at least 40 grams of fiber per day?

....

....

....

....

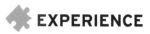 **EXPERIENCE**

Breakfast revisited: What creative breakfast options can you think of?

> "We are indeed much more than what we eat, but what we eat can nevertheless help us to be much more than what we are."
>
> [Adelle Davis]

Breakfast is the first meal of the day and your chance to set up for a day of great food choices. A good breakfast can keep you feeling sustained well into the day, so you are less likely to reach for unhealthy snacks or make poor meal choices later in the day.

› Aim to include a whole grain food to ensure your breakfast is substantial. A whole grain cereal-based food, such as whole grain wheat cereal, oats, 7-grain cereal, whole grain, bread, quinoa or even brown rice, can be a great source of long-lasting energy for the day.

› Breakfast is a great time to eat fruit. It can provide sweetness and a burst of flavor to subtly flavored grains. Fresh, dried and pureed fruits can be used to add variety.

› Different types of plant-based milks have different flavors. Try soy, rice, almond and oat milks with whole grain cereals for added variety. Make sure to choose plant-based milks fortified with vitamin B12.

› Think outside the box. Our idea of what is a "breakfast" food is often determined by culture, rather than nutritional factors. A healthy meal is a healthy meal, whether you choose to eat it at breakfast, lunch or dinner.

› Plan for variety. Weekdays can be a rush getting out of the house to begin the workday. Have some quick healthy breakfast options in mind for when you know you'll be short on time. On those days with more time, treat yourself to more elaborate options to keep things interesting.

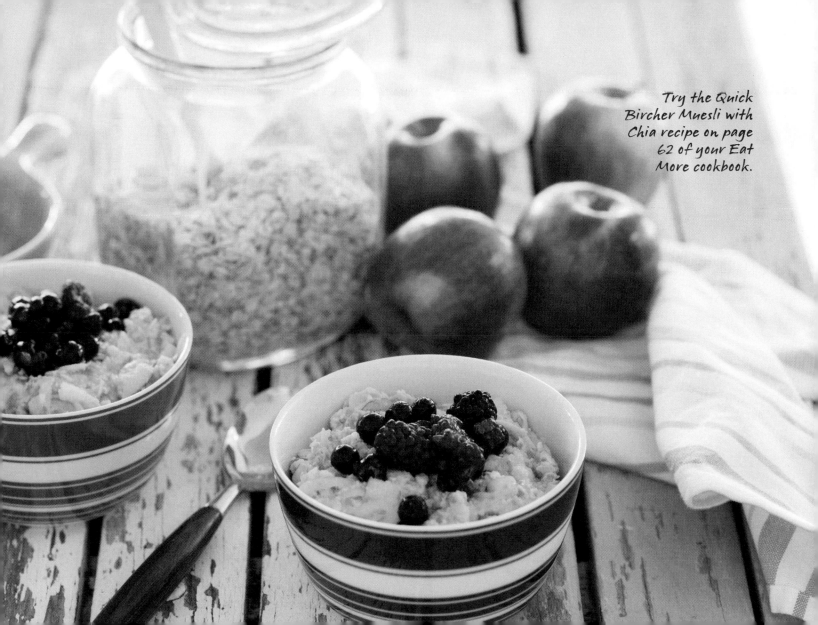

Try the Quick Bircher Muesli with Chia recipe on page 62 of your Eat More cookbook.

Fiber All-Stars:
The Top 10 Fiber Foods

1. Legumes are an amazing food, full of fiber, protein and good carbohydrates, and low in fat. They are a nutrition powerhouse and should be a key part of any plant-based meal. Legumes such as navy beans, lentils, black beans and kidney beans contain between 6 and 10 grams of fiber per half cup.

2. Whole grain cereals are the perfect example of the difference processing and fiber can make to a food. Refined cereal products can offer little nutritional value, while whole grains are the optimal source of slow-release fuel for our body. Whole grains such as whole wheat, quinoa, oats and brown rice contain anywhere between 4 and 8 grams of fiber per cup.

3. Chia seeds and flaxseeds are a concentrated source of fiber, containing 8 to 11 grams of fiber per 1 ounce (30g) of seeds. Purchase whole flaxseeds and grind just before eating for maximum benefit.

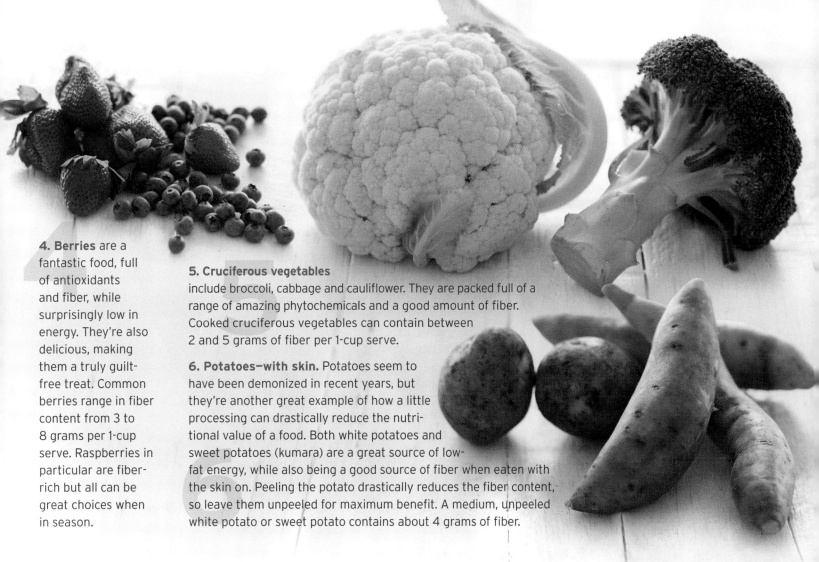

4. Berries are a fantastic food, full of antioxidants and fiber, while surprisingly low in energy. They're also delicious, making them a truly guilt-free treat. Common berries range in fiber content from 3 to 8 grams per 1-cup serve. Raspberries in particular are fiber-rich but all can be great choices when in season.

5. Cruciferous vegetables include broccoli, cabbage and cauliflower. They are packed full of a range of amazing phytochemicals and a good amount of fiber. Cooked cruciferous vegetables can contain between 2 and 5 grams of fiber per 1-cup serve.

6. Potatoes—with skin. Potatoes seem to have been demonized in recent years, but they're another great example of how a little processing can drastically reduce the nutritional value of a food. Both white potatoes and sweet potatoes (kumara) are a great source of low-fat energy, while also being a good source of fiber when eaten with the skin on. Peeling the potato drastically reduces the fiber content, so leave them unpeeled for maximum benefit. A medium, unpeeled white potato or sweet potato contains about 4 grams of fiber.

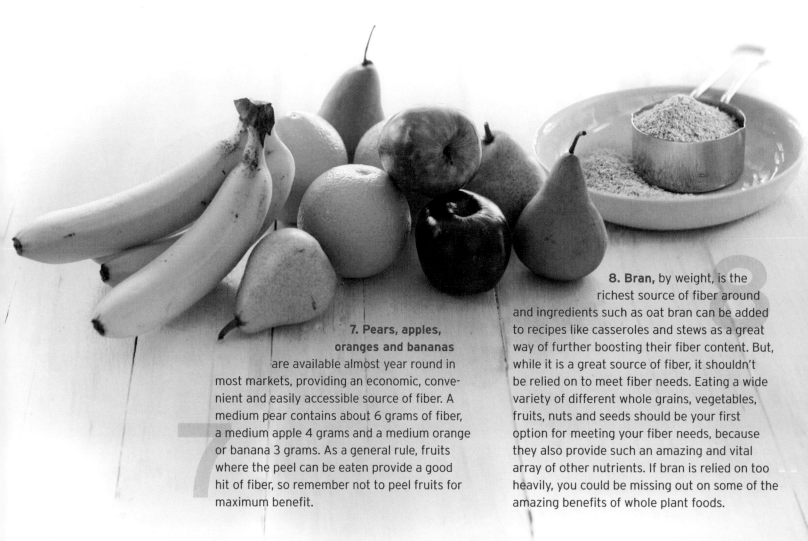

7. Pears, apples, oranges and bananas are available almost year round in most markets, providing an economic, convenient and easily accessible source of fiber. A medium pear contains about 6 grams of fiber, a medium apple 4 grams and a medium orange or banana 3 grams. As a general rule, fruits where the peel can be eaten provide a good hit of fiber, so remember not to peel fruits for maximum benefit.

8. Bran, by weight, is the richest source of fiber around and ingredients such as oat bran can be added to recipes like casseroles and stews as a great way of further boosting their fiber content. But, while it is a great source of fiber, it shouldn't be relied on to meet fiber needs. Eating a wide variety of different whole grains, vegetables, fruits, nuts and seeds should be your first option for meeting your fiber needs, because they also provide such an amazing and vital array of other nutrients. If bran is relied on too heavily, you could be missing out on some of the amazing benefits of whole plant foods.

As a rule, high-fiber foods are not very energy-dense, making them great low-energy foods to base your meals around. There are two notable exceptions to this rule; avocado and nuts are energy-dense foods that are also great sources of fiber. This doesn't make them unhealthy, but be aware that they can be easier to overeat than many other plant foods.

9. Avocado is an unusual fruit as it is higher in fat than carbohydrate and protein. However, a medium avocado also contains about 14 grams of fiber, as well as being a source of B vitamins, vitamin E and potassium. Some people find avocado can be great as a spread instead of butter when transitioning toward a lower-fat diet.

10. Nuts can pack a potent dose of fiber in a small package, with walnuts, peanuts and almonds containing between 2 to 4 grams per ounce. They also pack a punch when it comes to energy density, to get the greatest benefit, limit nuts to about 1 ounce (or a small handful) a day.

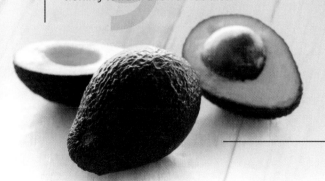

Low-fiber versus high-fiber foods

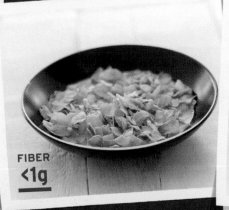

FIBER
<1g

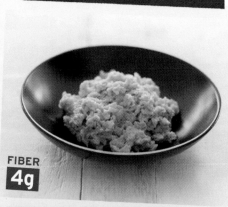

FIBER
4g

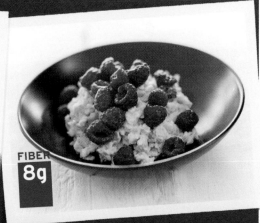

FIBER
8g

LOW FIBER	FIBER	HIGHER FIBER	FIBER	FIBER MAXIMIZER	FIBER
Corn flakes (1 cup)	<1g	**Oatmeal/porridge** (1 cup)	4g	**Oatmeal topped with raspberries** (✢ cup)	8g
Mashed potato (1 cup/7.5oz/210g)	3g	**Baked potato with skin** (7.5oz/210g)	4.5g	**Baked potato with skin topped with chili beans** (✢ cup)	10g
Cheeseburger (regular patty, cheese white bun, condiments)	3g	**Tofu Vegie Burger** (*Simple, Tasty, Good*, page 74)	4g	**Tofu Vegie Burger with salad on a mixed grain roll**	7g

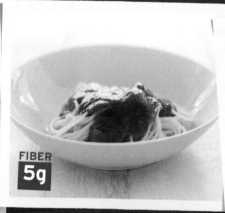

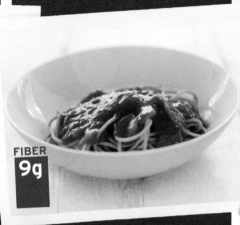

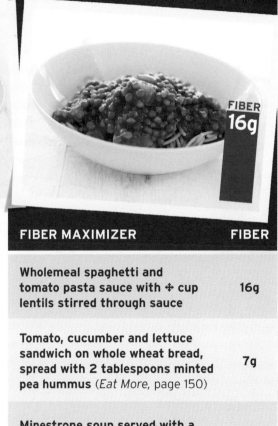

FIBER
5g

FIBER
9g

FIBER
16g

LOW FIBER	FIBER
Spaghetti and tomato pasta sauce (1 cup spaghetti, ⬩ cup sauce)	**5g**
Ham sandwich on white bread	**1.5g**
Canned tomato soup (2 cups)	**3g**

HIGHER FIBER	FIBER
Wholemeal spaghetti and tomato pasta sauce	**9g**
Tomato, cucumber and lettuce sandwich on whole wheat bread	**5g**
Minestrone soup (*Eat More*, page 51, 1 serve)	**5g**

FIBER MAXIMIZER	FIBER
Wholemeal spaghetti and tomato pasta sauce with ⬩ cup lentils stirred through sauce	**16g**
Tomato, cucumber and lettuce sandwich on whole wheat bread, spread with 2 tablespoons minted pea hummus (*Eat More*, page 150)	**7g**
Minestrone soup served with a toasted slice of whole wheat bread	**7g**

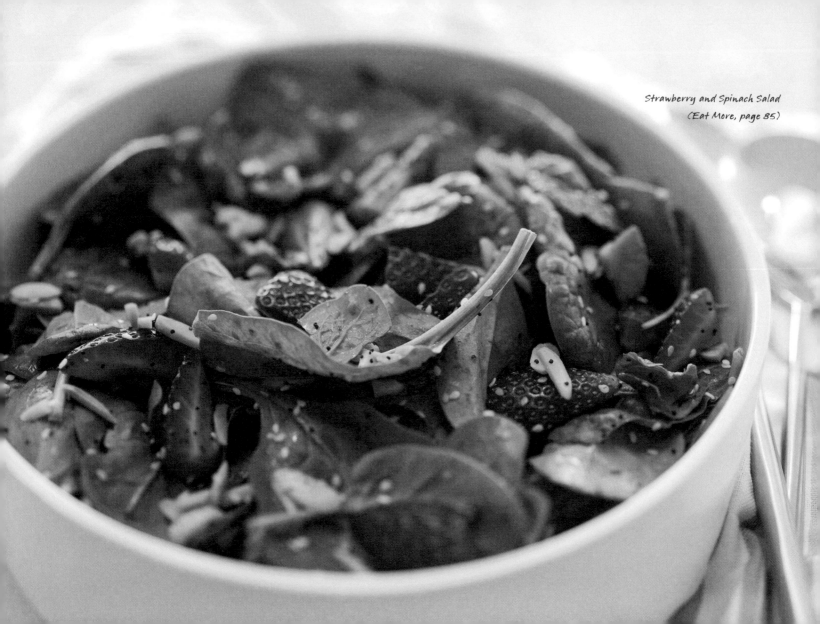

Strawberry and Spinach Salad
(Eat More, page 85)

High-fiber meal plan

	MEAL PLAN 1	FIBER	MEAL PLAN 2	FIBER	MEAL PLAN 3	FIBER
Breakfast	**Quick Bircher Muesli** (*Eat More*, page 62) **and an apple**	13g	**Homemade Baked Beans** (*Eat More*, page 55), **1 slice of whole wheat toast and a pear**	15g	**Oatmeal topped with raspberries and a banana**	11g
Lunch	**Roast Pepper and Pumpkin Soup** (*Eat More*, page 98), **1 slice of whole wheat bread and a pear**	17g	**Lentil Shepherd's Pie** (*Eat More*, page 128) **served with Cabbage and Pineapple Salad** (*Eat More*, page 81), **finishing with a banana**	16g	**Baked potato topped with chili beans, followed by a pear**	16g
Supper/ Dinner	**Lentil and Sesame Rissoles** (*Eat More*, page 120), **served with Strawberry and Spinach Salad** (*Eat More*, page 85)	13g	**Split Pea and Cumin Hotpot** (*Eat More*, page 48), **with 1 slice of whole wheat bread**	12g	**Wholemeal spaghetti and tomato pasta sauce with ⅓ cup lentils stirred through sauce**	11g
TOTAL FIBER		**43g**		**43g**		**38g**

All values rounded to closest 0.5g. Nutrition values taken from USDA nutrient database unless taken from CHIP *Eat More* recipe book or *Simple, Tasty, Good*.

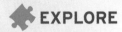 **EXPLORE**

Read *Learn More*, Chapter Five

› In what way can fiber be a "friend"?

....

....

....

....

....

› What should you look for to help in choosing foods with high fiber?

....

....

....

....

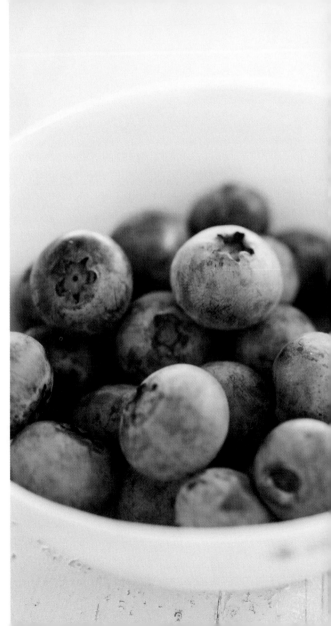

› While perhaps sometimes necessary, why are whole plant-based foods more advantageous than taking supplements?

....

....

·

....

....

....

....

....

....

› What is the function of the good bacteria "probiotics" in the digestive process?

....

....

....

....

....

....

....

....

› Think of your favorite three meals. What could you substitute in or add to these meals to increase their fiber content?

1 ....

....

2 ....

....

3 ....

....

....

SHARE

Bake a delicious treat for family or friends—try the Carrot Cake recipe on page 171 of *Eat More*.

Until the next session, keep notes of your weekly changes on page 155, recording what you change, and what has worked well—or not so well—for you in making these changes.

Session Seven

Disarming Diabetes

🧩 DISCOVER

› What three things have you learned about diabetes?

....

....

....

....

› Why is diabetes such a major problem as a disease?

....

....

....

....

"With good lifestyle choices— particularly healthy diet and regular activity— the risks of developing type 2 diabetes can be dramatically reduced."

› There has been a 900 per cent increase in diabetes in some age groups since World War II. What do you think accounts for this?

....

....

> What percentage of people with type 2 diabetes does Dr James Anderson suggest could normalize their blood sugar levels and get off medication within weeks, if they change their diet?

....

....

....

....

....

> What can you do to help prevent or improve type 2 diabetes?

....

....

....

....

....

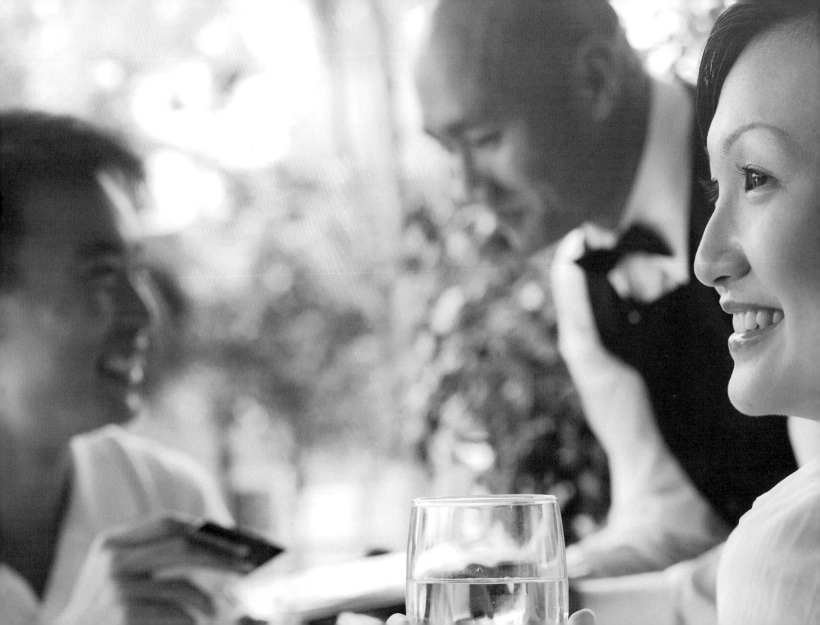

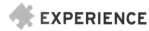 **EXPERIENCE**

Enjoy a healthy restaurant, cafe or take-away meal, choosing the venue and making the menu choice using the optimal diet principles.

Strategies for healthy eating out

Food plays an incredibly important role in our social lives. It's often the way we celebrate and connect with friends and family. Strategies for eating out are important because you don't want to abandon your healthy lifestyle, but you also shouldn't miss out on these important opportunities to build on great relationships with the ones you love.

> Think about what styles of foods favor healthy choices—and aim for them. For example, fast-food restaurants are probably not going to offer as many good options as a restaurant basing their menu on a traditional cuisine.

> Look at the whole menu. For example, just because something is listed as a side salad doesn't mean it has to accompany a hulking main dish. Try ordering a couple of healthy looking salads or "starters" instead of a main meal.

> Watch out for sauces. Rich sauces or dressings can turn a healthy meal into a questionable one. Don't be afraid to ask if a meal or salad is dressed with anything and don't be afraid to ask for it without it. Well-prepared, fresh foods can be bursting with amazing flavors that don't need to be covered up by dressings.

> Remember, you can always ask for something different to the menu. Would you like that pasta dish without cheese? Just ask—most restaurants are happy to make changes to suit your needs.

> Don't forget about drinks. Alcoholic drinks, juices and soda/soft drinks can add up to a lot of calories and sugar by the end of a meal. Most restaurants provide water at your table free of charge, making it the cheapest and healthiest option when eating out.

> The dessert menus often tempt even the strongest wills. Some restaurants offer fruit salad or fruit platters, which can be a good choice. If the menu seems devoid of good options, why not finish the meal relaxing with friends over a nice cup of caffeine-free herbal tea?

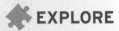 **EXPLORE**

Read *Learn More,* Chapter Seven

› What are the three types of diabetes? What percentage of people with diabetes have type 2 diabetes?

....

....

....

....

....

› What constitutes a diagnosis of type 2 diabetes?

....

....

....

....

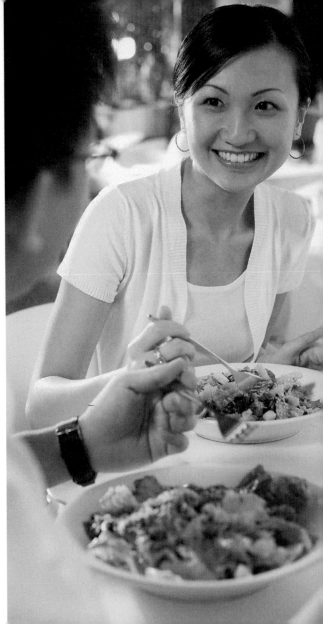

> Higher risk of type 2 diabetes is associated with what lifestyle behaviors?

....

....

....

....

> How does the "Optimal Lifestyle" protect from diabetes?

....

....

....

> Why do you need the supervision of your doctor or physician in making this kind of lifestyle change, particularly if you have a pre-existing condition like diabetes?

....

....

....

....

....

....

....

SHARE

Tell your CHIP group about a local venue—restaurant or café—where you have enjoyed a healthy meal.

Until the next session, keep notes of your weekly changes on page 155, recording what you change, and what has worked well—or not so well—for you in making these changes.

The Heart of the Matter—Heart Health

✦ DISCOVER

> What three things have you learned about cholesterol and heart health?

> Have you been surprised by your blood cholesterol results, particularly now that you know more about cholesterol and what it is?

....

....

....

....

....

....

....

....

....

....

....

....

"Health is the thing that makes you feel that now is the best time of the year."

[Franklin P Adams]

› How does the body make cholesterol?

....

....

....

....

....

....

› What is the good news about the link between diet and cholesterol levels in the blood?

....

....

....

....

› What role does nitric oxide play in the health of the circulatory system?

....

....

....

....

....

› What are the most significant steps you can take to lower your cholesterol levels?

....

....

....

....

EXPERIENCE

Strategies for healthy eating while traveling

The key to successful lifestyle change is that it needs to be sustainable, so it's important to have some strategies to deal with common situations, like traveling. Just because you go on a holiday, it doesn't mean you have to leave your healthy lifestyle at home, but it also doesn't mean you have to spend all your time chained to the kitchen.

› Research where you're traveling to. A whole range of websites and tourist guidebooks can help you scope out restaurants in the area to see which ones might have better choices.

› If you're traveling by plane, check what menu options are available. Most airlines have options covering dietary choices for a range of health and religious reasons.

› Make the buffet your friend. Many hotels have buffets available at meal times, particularly breakfast. While they often have many poor options, they usually also have a lot of good ones available. Use the buffet as a chance not to be bound by menus. Fill your plate with fruits, vegetables, salads and whole grains.

› Make the best out of every situation. Sometimes on long trips, we can find ourselves in places with poor access to good food. We've all been in that situation when it seems like the only options around are fast-food restaurants. The key is not to use that as an excuse to make poor choices. Even on a fast-food menu, there's a continuum of choices from best to worst. If you find yourself in this situation, make the best choice available and look forward to your next meal.

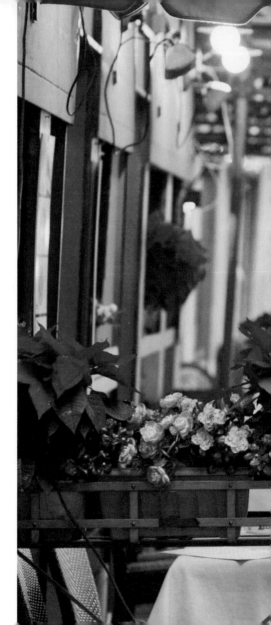

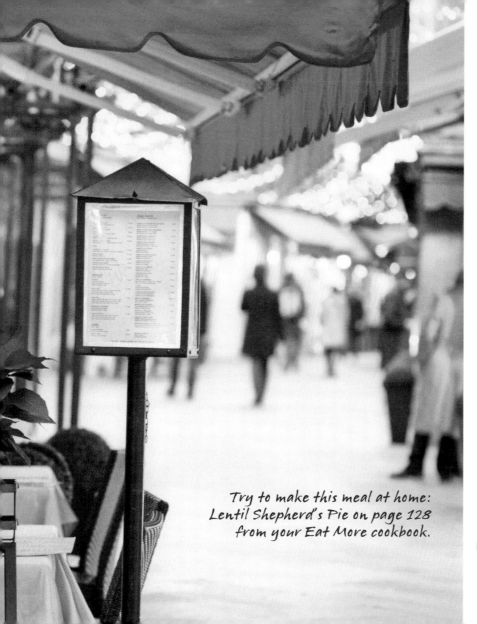

Try to make this meal at home: Lentil Shepherd's Pie on page 128 from your Eat More cookbook.

Some common sources of cholesterol

FOOD	CHOLESTEROL (mg)
Milk, Skim (1 cup)	**5**
Cottage Cheese (1 cup)	**36**
Ice Cream (1 cup)	**58**
Chedder Cheese (1 ounce/30g)	**30**
Beef (3 ounces/90g)	**59**
Salmon (3 ounces/90g)	**65**
Pork (3 ounces/90g)	**72**
Chicken (3 ounces/90g)	**76**
Shrimp (3 ounces/90g)	**113**
1 Egg Yolk	**184**
Liver–lamb (3 ounces/90g)	**314**

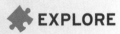 **EXPLORE**

Read *Learn More*, Chapter Six

> Does your family have a "history" of heart disease? What lifestyle factors may have contributed to this "history"?

....

....

....

....

> What is the difference between HDL and LDL cholesterol?

....

....

....

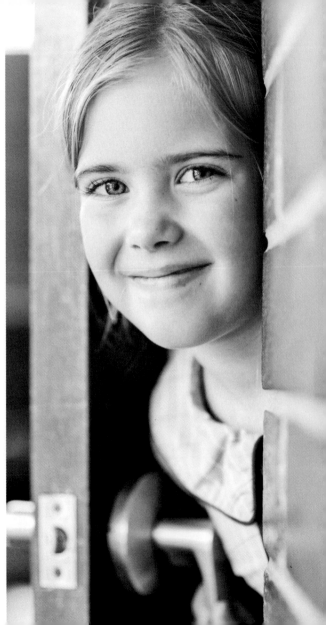

› What is the relationship between fat in foods eaten and blood cholesterol levels?

....

....

....

› How would you explain what "blood pressure" is to a class of school children?

....

....

....

....

› Of the six lifestyle factors for high blood pressure, what opportunities do you have to make improvements?

....

....

....

....

› Why can some processed foods be high in sodium?

....

....

....

....

SHARE

Share with your CHIP group ideas on how to prepare tasty meals with less salt/sodium. You can find some suggestions on pages 12-15 of your *Eat More* cookbook.

Until the next session, keep notes of your weekly changes on page 155, recording what you change, and what has worked well—or not so well—for you in making these changes.

Controlling Blood Pressure and Discovering Protein

🧩 DISCOVER:

› What three things have you learned about the contributors to high blood pressure?

....

....

....

....

....

....

....

› In what ways does high blood pressure affect the health of the heart?

....

....

....

....

....

....

....

"A man too busy to take care of his health is like a mechanic too busy to take care of his tools."

[Spanish Proverb]

› Why is salt such a significant contributor to high blood pressure?

....

....

....

....

› Do you have concerns about possible nutritional deficiencies in a plant-based diet? What are they?

....

....

....

....

› Why is it surprising to learn that most of us are unlikely to lack protein in our diet?

....

....

....

....

› How does a plant-based diet provide adequate protein?

....

....

....

....

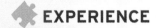 **EXPERIENCE**

Reduce salt intake

Salt is one of those components of food that can often be forgotten. It doesn't contribute to weight gain, but its link to the silent but high-risk condition of high blood pressure makes it important for us to watch our intake. On top of this, the vast majority of salt found in Western diets is hidden in processed foods—where it is listed on nutrition panels under "sodium"—rather than added at the table, making it even more important to have strategies for reducing salt in the diet.

› While an optimal diet is based around whole plant foods, some pre-packaged foods, such as bread, can be a valuable part of a healthy diet. When selecting packaged foods, compare the available options and choose the variety with the lowest sodium content. Some people find a useful rule to follow is to only choose foods that have less sodium than calories per serve. For example, a food with 300 calories (1250kJ) would need to contain less than 300mg of sodium.

› Breads can be a major source of sodium in the diet. Salt is used in the baking process because it plays a role in the rising process and contributes to the color of that distinctive brown crust. Read the labels and compare breads to find the lowest sodium variety that meets your needs.

› Sauces and other condiments such as relishes are often high in sodium, as the salt is used to preserve the main ingredients. Become a label detective when it comes to sauces and dressings and only choose the lowest sodium options available. Better yet, opt for low-salt homemade versions where possible. Make your own low-salt sauces by puréeing cooked tomatoes—or "Low Sodium" or "No Added Salt" canned tomatoes—with herbs such as basil or oregano.

> Watch out for canned foods. Like some sauces, many canned foods contain significant amounts of added salt to help preserve them. Canned beans and vegetables can be convenient pantry staples, just make sure to choose varieties with the lowest sodium content and rinse well after opening to get rid of any excess.

> Be careful of stocks. Liquid stocks and powders provide a concentrated source of flavor, but also a good deal of sodium. Where possible, flavor recipes with fresh ingredients and if using a stock, choose one with as little sodium as possible.

> Use herbs and spices to flavor dishes instead of adding salt. Some herbs will work better with certain foods. Check out page 12-15 of *Eat More* for a handy guide to combining flavors.

> Get the best-quality food you have access to. Look for fruits and vegetables in season and fresh. High-quality seasonal produce is packed with natural flavor.

> Use small amounts of strongly flavored ingredients to bring meals to life. For example, a squeeze of lemon or lime juice over a salad or through a stir-fry can completely change a meal, providing a burst of flavor.

Check for hidden salt

Many different forms of salt are found in food products, often with different names.
Read through the ingredients list to identify hidden sources of salt, such as:

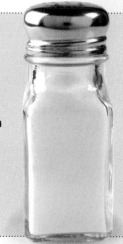

- Sodium
- Monosodium glutamate or MSG
- Sodium bicarbonate
- Sodium lactate
- Sodium ascorbate
- Sodium metabisulphite

- Sodium nitrate
- Sodium citrate
- Celery salt
- Sodium phosphate
- Meat or yeast extract
- Hydrolysed vegetable or meat protein

- Stock cubes
- Vegetable or chicken or beef stock
- Baking powder or soda
- Rock salt
- Vegetable salt

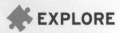 **EXPLORE**

Read *Learn More*, Chapter Nine

> What is the most significant nutritional myth that has been challenged by what you have learned on your CHIP journey?

....

....

....

....

> What are the two main types of bone cells and what do they do? How do they interact with calcium in our diet?

....

....

....

....

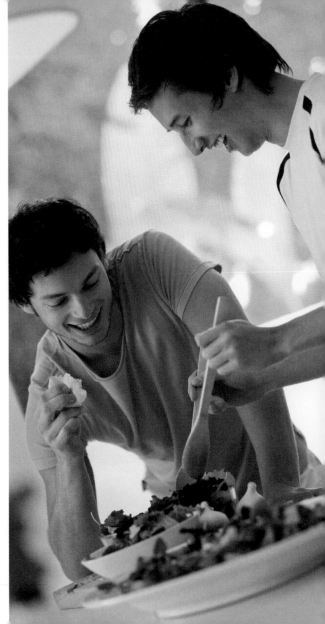

> What is the best way of getting vitamin D and what does this important vitamin do for us?

....

....

....

....

> How can a vegetarian ensure the absorption of sufficient iron from their diet?

....

....

....

....

> What is your favorite recipe using legumes?

....

....

....

> When should we be most careful about our levels of vitamin B12?

....

....

....

....

Until the next session, keep notes of your weekly changes on page 156, recording what you change, and what has worked well—or not so well—for you in making these changes.

SHARE

Prepare a dish based on legumes for friends and family members. See *Eat More* pages 48, 55, 56, 123, 124, 127, 128, 131, 135 and 138 for inspiration.

Session Ten

Bone Health Essentials

🧩 DISCOVER

› What three things have you learned?

....

....

....

› What are the factors that determine bone health?

....

....

....

› Were you surprised to learn that osteoporosis and associated hip fractures were more frequent in populations that consume a higher amount of dairy products? Explain.

....

....

....

....

"Our health always seems much more valuable after we lose it."

› What are the benefits of resistance training?

....

....

....

....

› How can you incorporate resistance training into your everyday schedule?

....

....

....

› What are some plant foods that are good sources of calcium?

....

....

....

....

Calcium in common plant foods

FOOD	CALCIUM (mg)
Soy milk (fortified with calcium) (1 cup)	300
Soybeans (1 cup, cooked)	175
Collard greens (½ cup chopped, boiled)	133
Tofu, set with calcium sulfate (½ cup)	126
Kale (1 cup chopped, boiled)	94
Sesame seeds (1 tablespoon)	88
Almonds (1 oz)	75
Orange (1 medium)	60
Rhubarb (½ cup chopped, raw)	53
Baked beans (½ cup, canned)	43
Cabbage (1 cup shredded, cooked)	36
Broccoli (1 cup chopped, cooked)	31
Dates (2, pitted)	30

EXPERIENCE

> Create a resistance training schedule and give it a go!

Resistance exercising

Resistance exercises can be of great benefit to people of all ages, but become especially important as we get older. They should be thought of as practical exercises, because the benefits of them can really be seen in everyday life. Resistance exercises help keep our muscles and bones strong, so we can power through the everyday tasks that some people find harder with age.

> **START OUT EASY:** There's no point finding the hardest resistance or the biggest weight you can and hurting yourself. Start out easy and work your way up to greater resistance.

> **REST:** Some muscle soreness is normal when starting new activities and can be a sign that you are responding to the training. But soreness shouldn't be so bad it prevents you from doing day-to-day tasks. Remember to include rest days in between resistance training the same part of the body so your muscles have time to recover.

> **AIM FOR VARIETY:** To get the greatest benefits out of resistance training, it's important to train all major muscle groups of the body. Think about something simple, like picking up a box from the ground and putting it on a high shelf. You use your legs to crouch down and lift the box from the ground, keeping your core muscles tense to keep the strain off your back, before using your chest, shoulders and arms to place the box up on the shelf. Everyday tasks use your whole body, so it makes sense to exercise the whole body.

Performed regularly, strength-building exercises are tremendously helpful for reducing fall-related injuries.

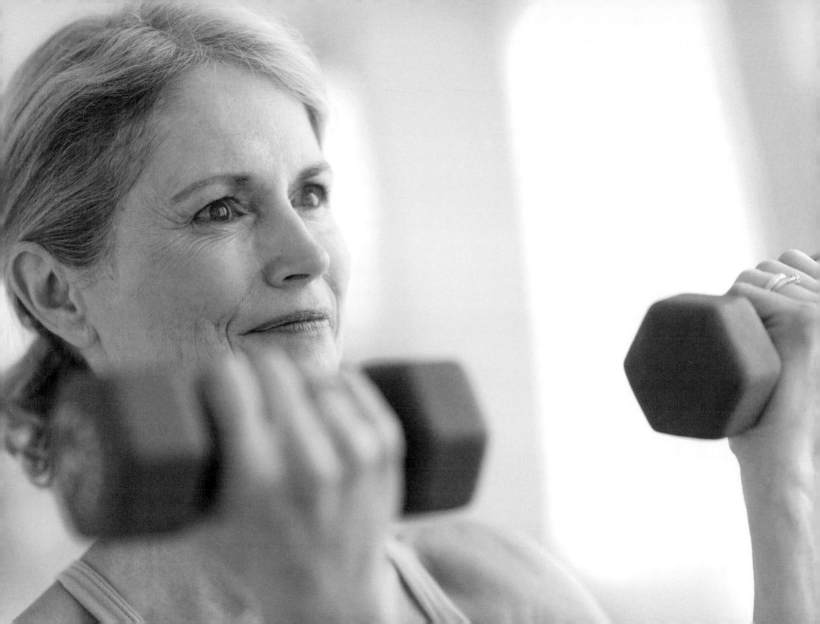

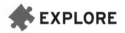 **EXPLORE**

Read *Learn More,* Chapter Eleven

› What does is mean to "move naturally"?

....

....

....

....

....

....

....

....

....

› How does regular exercise boost vitality?

....

....

....

....

› How does exercise affect appetite?

....

....

....

....

> Record on the clock the hours you sit during a normal week day.

> What household items can you use for exercise at home?

....

....

....

....

....

....

Until the next session, keep notes of your weekly changes on page 156, recording what you change, and what has worked well—or not so well—for you in making these changes.

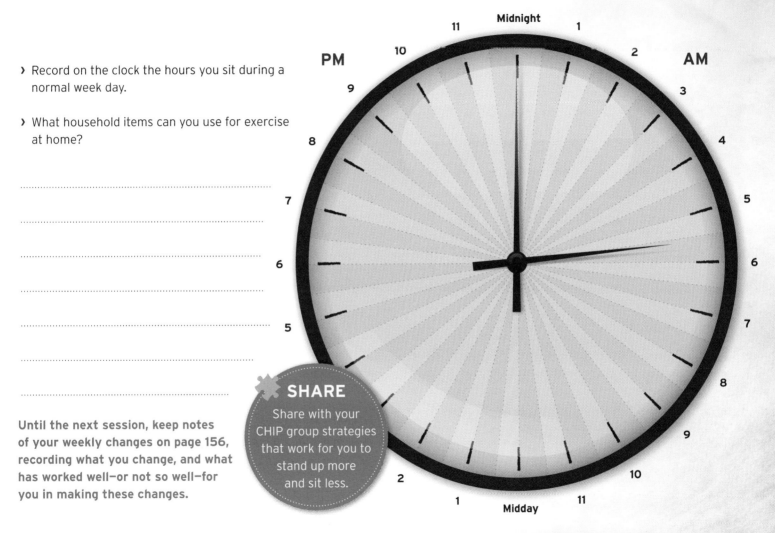

SHARE
Share with your CHIP group strategies that work for you to stand up more and sit less.

Session Eleven

Cancer Prevention

DISCOVER

› What three things have you learned?

....

....

....

....

....

....

....

› Is there a link between cancer and diet? In what ways might a whole food plant-based diet be protective from cancer?

....

....

....

› What are the links between cancer and lifestyle?

....

....

....

"To get rich never risk your health. For it is the truth that health is the wealth of wealth."

[Richard Baker]

› What steps can you take to reduce your risk of cancer?

....

....

....

....

....

....

....

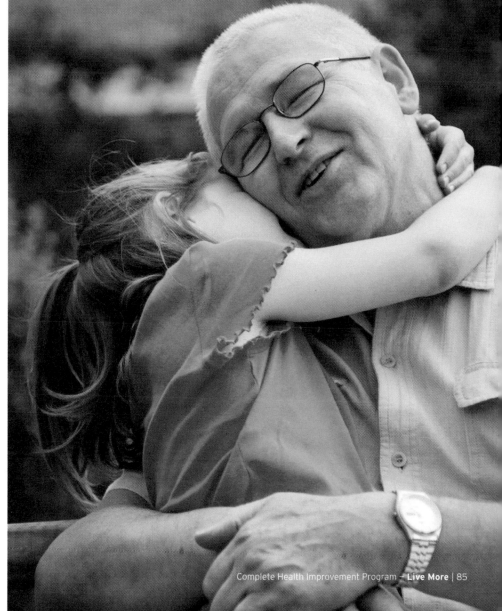

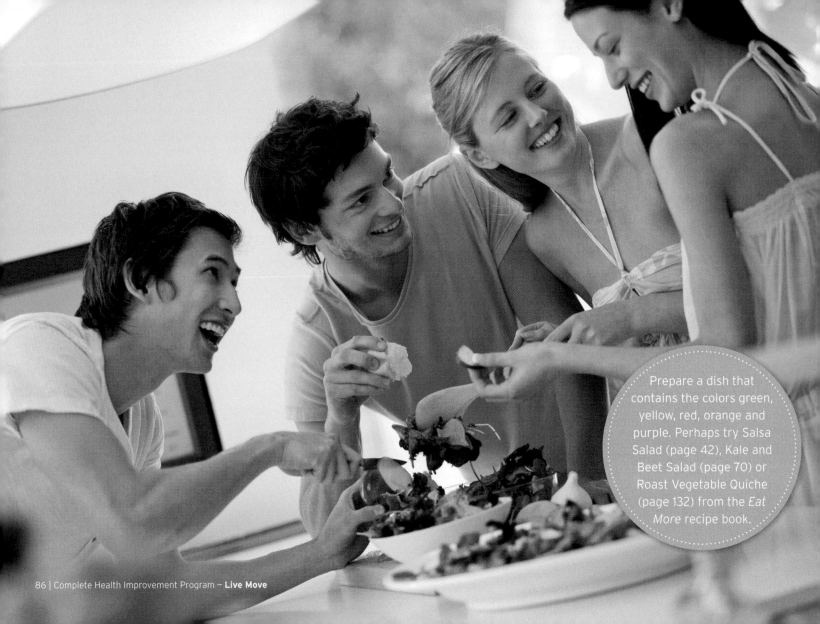

Prepare a dish that contains the colors green, yellow, red, orange and purple. Perhaps try Salsa Salad (page 42), Kale and Beet Salad (page 70) or Roast Vegetable Quiche (page 132) from the *Eat More* recipe book.

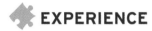 **EXPERIENCE**

Eat a rainbow

Have you ever been stuck in a food rut, when you seem to eat the same five meals over and over again? Not only does it get boring, but it also means you could be missing out on valuable nutrients. This can especially be a real danger when making a dietary change, when everything is new and can be a bit overwhelming. Eating a wide variety of foods is important because no one or two foods contain all the different nutrients we need to live happy, healthy lives. Research has shown that different colored plant foods contain different types of phytonutrients that you don't want to miss out on.

> **Pick one new food every week and try to incorporate it into a meal.** Explore the fresh food section of your supermarket and take a risk—you never know what might be your new favorite food.

> **Do some research.** This doesn't have to mean scouring every cookbook you can find, but ask friends and family or look on the internet for the best way to cook a particular food. The way a food is cooked or prepared could be the difference between a bland pile of mush and a delicious explosion of tastes and textures.

> **Aim to include at least three different colors in every meal.** Not only will it help with getting a wide range of foods across the day, it will keep your meals looking vibrant and inviting.

Research has shown that different colored plant foods contain different types of phytonutrients that you don't want to miss out on.

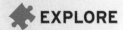 **EXPLORE**

Read *Learn More,* Chapter Eight

> What are the eight recommendations that the World Cancer Research Fund makes?

1 ....

....

2 ....

....

3 ....

....

4 ....

....

5 ....

....

6 ....

....

7 ....

....

8 ....

....

> Which of these recommendations do you need to incorporate into your lifestyle?

....

....

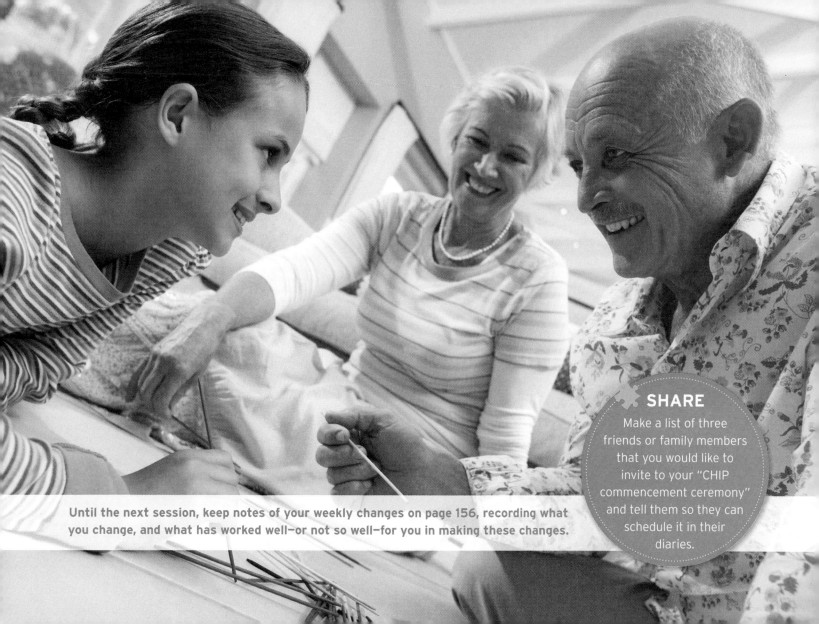

Until the next session, keep notes of your weekly changes on page 156, recording what you change, and what has worked well—or not so well—for you in making these changes.

SHARE

Make a list of three friends or family members that you would like to invite to your "CHIP commencement ceremony" and tell them so they can schedule it in their diaries.

Understanding Your Results and Taking Action

❇ DISCOVER

› What three things have you learned?

....

....

....

....

....

....

Our beliefs serve as the reference for how we feel, then those feelings drive our behaviors.

› What is your reaction to the results which you received today?

....

....

....

....

› What was your reaction to the story of Mavis Lindgren? Every journey begins with the first step. What is your next step?

....

....

....

....

› What destination do you want to arrive at?

....

....

....

....

....

› Are there ways in which you can implement more of the CHIP lifestyle?

....

....

....

....

....

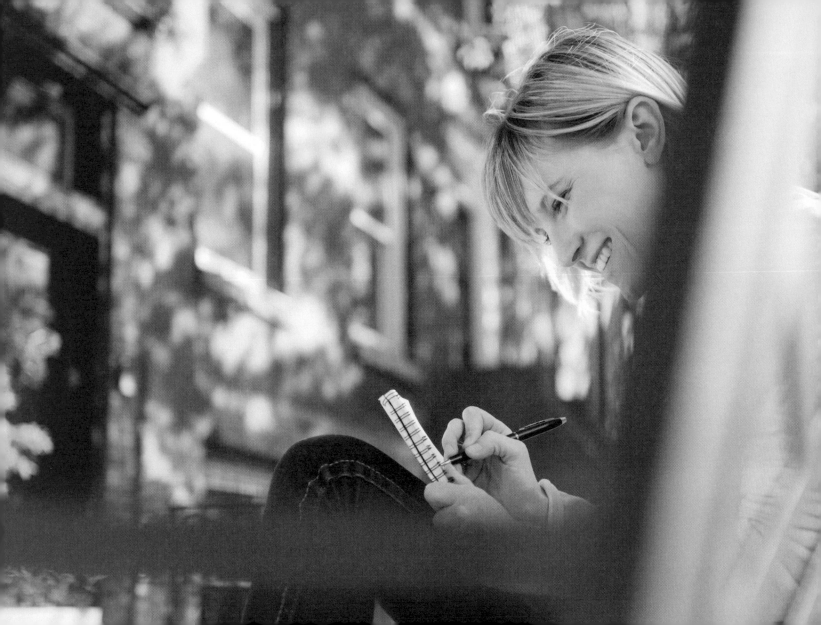

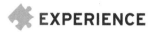 **EXPERIENCE**

> **Write down a SMART goal in one area of lifestyle change that you need to make.**

Goal setting and goal getting

By setting SMART goals, it is easier to identify how to succeed. When we encounter roadblocks, these goals provide a great way of breaking them down and moving past them.

> **Take goals seriously.** Sometimes it can be easy to say, "I'll do that next time"–but next time never comes. Holding ourselves accountable for our goals isn't always easy, but by coming up with goals that are relevant to what we want to achieve in our lives, we can find greater motivation to forget about "next time" and remember now.

> **Don't be afraid of failure.** SMART goals aren't about succeeding first time every time. If at first you don't succeed, maybe your goal needs to be broken down into a series of smaller goals. By going through the key points of your SMART goal, you might even find what you need to watch out for next time. Maybe your time frame wasn't long enough or perhaps you weren't specific enough in what you wanted to achieve.

> **No goal is too small.** Your goal could be as simple as "By the end of the next two weeks, I will be drinking one glass of water every morning before breakfast at least five times each week." Some of your goals might sound small or easy, but when you think about it, a healthy lifestyle is really a great benefit that comes from doing a lot of small, simple things.

SMART Goals and Action Plan

S
SPECIFIC

What are you going to achieve? What are the steps? This is where your Action Plan comes in handy!

M
MEASURABLE

How will you know that you have achieved your goal? How will others know?

A
ACHIEVABLE

What is needed to achieve this goal? Do you need anyone to help you achieve this goal?

R
RELEVANT

How does your goal relate to your health and wellbeing? What is the reason you would like to achieve this goal?

T
TIMELY

When do you plan to implement and reach your goal?

> Finally, it is a good idea to write the goal as if it is already a reality. Instead of writing "I would like to . . ." say "I am/I can . . ." We have provided an example below.

[*Define when you want to have achieved your goal.*]

[*The evidence: How you will know that your goal has been reached; your measures?*]

TODAY'S DATE	MY GOAL	WHEN?	RESULT
September 28	My fitness level has improved . . .	By the end of next month . . .	As evidenced by the fact that I can go for a 15 minute jog without stopping.

Action Plan: Steps to achieve your goal

ACTION STEPS *Consider specific strategies/methods*	HOW WILL I DO THIS? *Who is involved/ helping you; how often will you do it?*	WHEN WILL I DO THIS? *When will you do the things?*	WHAT DO I NEED TO DO THIS? *Equipment, schedule free time, certain ingredients, skills, knowledge, etc.*	HOW WILL I KNOW I HAVE DONE IT?
Go for a run (walk when necessary)	For 20 minutes with Katie	At lunch time at least 3 days during the work week	Take sport clothes and shoes to work, pack towel, shower gel, clean socks. Block out time and set automatic calendar reminders. Remind Katie to do the same. Take watch along on runs.	Circle days in calendar that I went for a run and note down the time I spent running. Count the days or weeks it took to reach my 15-minute running goal.

WOMEN

Small-boned: a wrist measurement of 5.25 inches (13 cm) or less.

Medium-boned: a wrist measurement between 5.25 to 6 inches (15 cm).

Large-boned: a wrist measurement of more than 6 inches.

WAIST MEASUREMENT	CHRONIC DISEASE RISK
Less than or equal to 31.5 inches (80 cm)	Low
31.5 to 34.5 inches (81 to 88 cm)	Increased
More than 34.5 inches (88 cm)	Greatly Increased

For more information on a healthy body weight, go to page 52 of *Learn More*

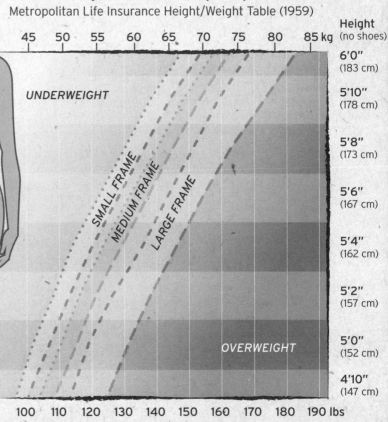

Ideal weights for women by body frame
Metropolitan Life Insurance Height/Weight Table (1959)

Height (no shoes)

45 50 55 60 65 70 75 80 85 kg

UNDERWEIGHT

SMALL FRAME
MEDIUM FRAME
LARGE FRAME

OVERWEIGHT

6'0" (183 cm)
5'10" (178 cm)
5'8" (173 cm)
5'6" (167 cm)
5'4" (162 cm)
5'2" (157 cm)
5'0" (152 cm)
4'10" (147 cm)

100 110 120 130 140 150 160 170 180 190 lbs

Weight includes one pound (450 grams) for ordinary indoor clothing.

MEN

Ideal weights for men by body frame

Metropolitan Life Insurance Height/Weight Table (1959)

Height
(no shoes)

6'4"	(193 cm)
6'2"	(188 cm)
6'0"	(183 cm)
5'10"	(178 cm)
5'8"	(173 cm)
5'6"	(167 cm)
5'4"	(162 cm)
5'2"	(157 cm)

55 60 65 70 75 80 85 90 95 kg

UNDERWEIGHT

SMALL FRAME

MEDIUM FRAME

LARGE FRAME

OVERWEIGHT

120 130 140 150 160 170 180 190 200 210 lbs

Weight includes one pound (450 grams) for ordinary indoor clothing.

Small-boned: a wrist measurement of anything less than 6 inches (15 cm)

Large-boned: a wrist measurement of anything more than 7 inches (17.5 cm)

CHRONIC DISEASE RISK	WAIST MEASUREMENT
Low	Less than or equal to 37 inches (94 cm)
Increased	37 to 40 inches (95 to 102 cm)
Greatly Increased	More than 40 inches (102 cm)

Australian Government (2003), "How to measure yourself," <http://www.measureup.gov.au/internet/abhi/publishing.nsf/Content/How+do+I+measure+myself-lp#measuring>.

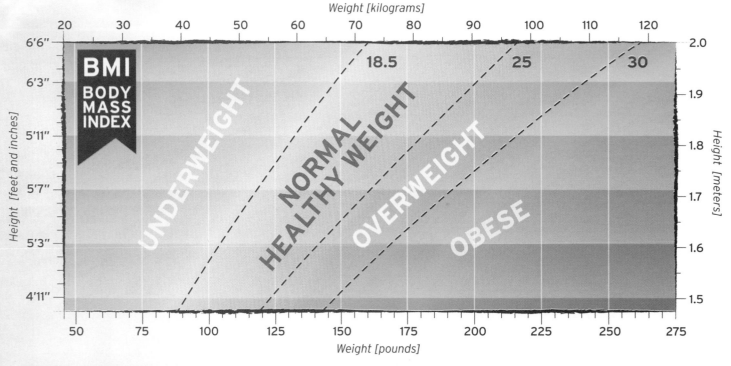

BMI
BODY MASS INDEX

Weight [kilograms]

UNDERWEIGHT

NORMAL HEALTHY WEIGHT

OVERWEIGHT

OBESE

18.5   25   30

Height [feet and inches]

Height [meters]

Weight [pounds]

YOUR BMI	Date	Result
Before CHIP		
Progress 1		
Progress 2		

BMI	Range of weight
Under 18.5	Underweight
18.5 to 24.9	Normal or healthy weight
25.0 to 29.9	Overweight
Over 30.0	Obese

Source: National Instute of Health

What is a healthy blood cholesterol level?

› **Less than 160 mg/dL (4.2mmol/L) total cholesterol**

› **Less than 90 mg/dL (2.3 mmol/L) for LDL cholesterol**

Remember, we can reduce the risk of developing atherosclerosis by reducing excess LDL cholesterol, as well as by reducing the risk of the LDL cholesterol being oxidized.

Researchers report a 1 to 3 per cent decrease in atherosclerosis risk for every 1 per cent decrease in blood LDL cholesterol. Results from CHIP studies indicate that it is possible to achieve reductions of up to 20 per cent in total cholesterol and LDL cholesterol, usually within four weeks, thereby reducing heart disease risk by up to 40 per cent.

For more information on on markers of heart health, go to pages 80-84 of *Learn More*

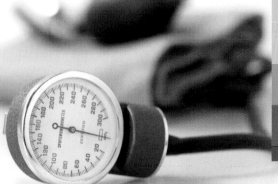

BLOOD PRESSURE READINGS

Blood pressure readings are a combination of two measurements:

› **Systolic** is the highest pressure against the arteries as the heart pumps. The normal systolic pressure is between 110 and 120mmHg.

› **Diastolic** is the pressure against the arteries as the heart relaxes and fills with blood. The normal diastolic pressure is between 70 and 80mmHg.

TARGET NUMBERS (mm Hg)

	Systolic		Diastolic
Normal	less than 120	and	less than 80
Pre-hypertension	120-139	or	80-89
High	140 and above	or	90 and above

Source: American Heart Association

*Heart Health: Why your blood lipid results may have gone up or down**

	HAS IT GONE UP?	HAS IT GONE DOWN?
Total Blood Cholesterol	You may have not progressed far enough along the healthy eating continuum to effect this, so consider further dietary and lifestyle changes. In particular, dietary sources of saturated and trans fats can negatively impact blood cholesterol levels. Including sufficient amounts of certain types of fiber found in whole plant foods can also help achieve healthy blood cholesterol levels. If you feel you have made a good effort to adopt a healthy lifestyle and these values have still increased or stayed the same, it is important to discuss other possible causes of increased blood cholesterol with your physician including familial hypercholesterolemia, familial hyperlipidemia, hypothyroidism and uncontrolled diabetes to help rule out any of these other potential causes. A reduction in cholesterol lowering medication between tests can also cause total and LDL cholesterol to remain the same or increase. Total cholesterol and LDL cholesterol may also not respond if the liver is or has been diseased.	If your total blood cholesterol was high to begin with, this is a desired result. This decrease in total blood cholesterol is a likely sign of how changes you have made to your diet and lifestyle have had a positive impact on your health. If your cholesterol levels were already desirable or low, discuss other possible causes of low cholesterol with your physician to rule out any undesirable causes.
LDL Cholesterol	You may have not progressed far enough along the healthy eating continuum to effect this, so consider further dietary and lifestyle changes. In particular, dietary sources of saturated and trans fats can negatively impact LDL cholesterol levels, while certain types of fiber found in whole plant foods can also help lower LDL levels.	If your LDL cholesterol was high to begin with, this is a desired result. This decrease in LDL cholesterol is a likely sign of how changes you have made to your diet and lifestyle have had a positive impact on your health.

HAS IT GONE UP?	HAS IT GONE DOWN?
If you feel you have made a good effort to adopt a healthy lifestyle and these values have still increased or stayed the same, it is important to discuss other possible causes of increased LDL cholesterol levels with your physician including familial LDL lipoproteinemia, glycogen storage diseases, hypothyroidism and chronic liver disease to help rule out any of these other potential causes.	If your LDL cholesterol levels were already desirable or low, discuss other possible causes of low LDL cholesterol with your physician to rule out any undesirable causes.

Triglycerides

You may have not progressed far enough along the healthy eating continuum to effect this, so consider further dietary and lifestyle changes. In particular, excess carbohydrates in the diet can result in a rise in triglycerides. Ensure meals are based on a balanced range of foods and are not too heavily reliant on refined carbohydrate foods.	If your triglycerides were high to begin with, this is a desired result. This decrease in triglycerides is a likely sign of how changes you have made to your diet and lifestyle have had a positive impact on your health.
If you feel you have made a good effort to adopt a healthy life-style and these values have still increased or stayed the same, it is important to discuss other possible causes of increased triglycerides with your physician including glycogen storage diseases, familial hypertriglyceridemia, hyperlipidemias, hypothyroidism, poorly controlled diabetes, nephrotic syndrome and chronic renal failure to help rule out any of these other potential causes.	If your triglycerides levels were already desirable or low, discuss other possible causes of low triglycerides with your physician to rule out any undesirable causes.

* This table is only intended as general information on factors which can commonly effect blood lipid levels. It is important to discuss all your test results with your physician.

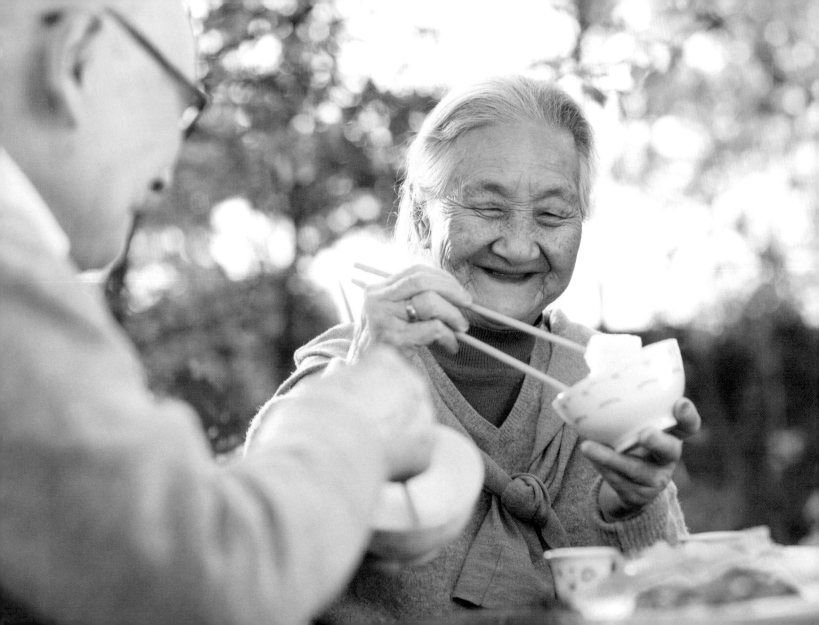

IDEAL BLOOD SUGAR LEVELS	FROM 60 TO 99 mg/dL

▲ Fasting plasma glucose from 60 to 99 mg/dL (3.3-5.5mmol/L).

PRE-DIABETES	BETWEEN 100 TO 125mg/dL

▲ Fasting plasma glucose of between 100 to 125mg/dL (5.6-6.9mmol/L)

DIABETES	GREATER THAN 125mg/dL	OR	GREATER THAN 200mg/dL AFTER GLUCOSE DRINK

▲ Two consecutive tests with fasting plasma glucose concentrations greater than or equal to 125mg/dL (7mmol/L) or greater than or equal to 200mg/dL (11.1mmol/L) 2 hours after a 2.65oz (75g) glucose drink.

What about HbA1c?

Hemoglobin A1c represents an average measurement of blood sugar over a few months.

A HbA1c of 5.6 per cent or less is normal.

The following are the results when the HbA1c is being used to diagnose diabetes:

Normal	Less than 5.7%
Pre-diabetes	5.7% to 6.4%
Diabetes	6.5% or higher

If you have diabetes, you and your doctor or nurse will discuss the correct range for you. For many people the goal is to keep your level at or below 6.5 -7 per cent.

For more information on blood glucose levels, go to page 96 of *Learn More.*

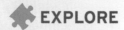 **EXPLORE**

Read *Learn More*, Chapter Twelve

› Explain the statement "You become what you believe."

....

....

....

....

....

› Have your taste buds changed while you have been doing the CHIP program? How?

....

....

....

....

....

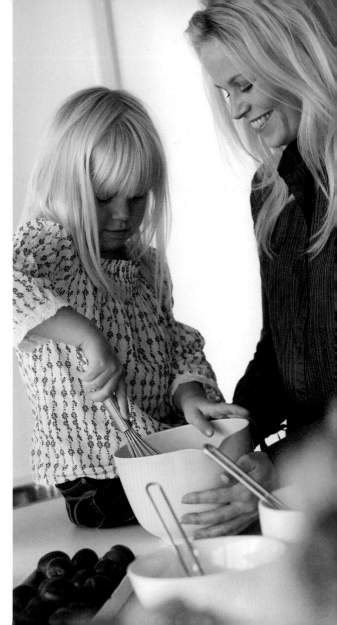

› What were the key factors that the National Weight Control Registry found for successfully maintaining weight loss?

....

....

....

....

....

› What are the five components of a SMART goal?

1 ....

2 ....

3 ....

4 ....

5 ....

› Outline why you will achieve success in applying your SMART goal to your lifestyle.

....

....

....

....

Until the next session, keep notes of your weekly changes on page 157, recording what you change, and what has worked well—or not so well—for you in making these changes.

SHARE

Share one of your SMART goals with a friend or family member and help them develop a SMART goal of their own.

Become What You Believe and Your DNA is Not Your Destiny

🧩 DISCOVER

› What three things have you learned?

....

....

....

....

....

....

› In what way do beliefs drive behavior?

....

....

....

....

....

....

"People don't have any difficulty motivating themselves to do whatever it takes to secure the source of their love or escape the source of their fear."

› Do you really believe that CHIP can work for you? Explain your answer.

....

....

....

....

....

› Do you really believe that you deserve CHIP success? Explain your answer.

....

....

....

....

› What gives you worth as an individual?

....

....

....

....

....

› Is your fate determined by genes? Explain your answer.

....

....

....

....

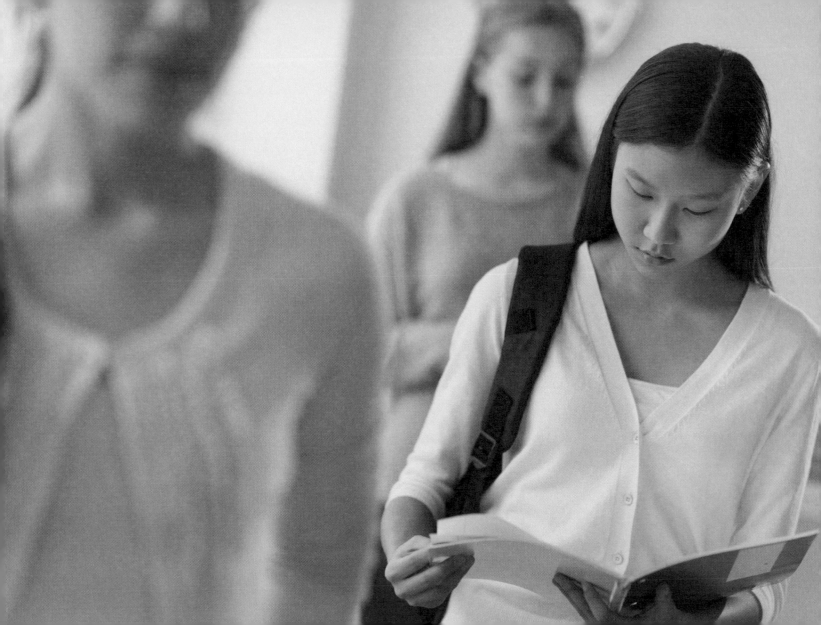

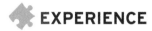 **EXPERIENCE**

Identify your roadblocks and barriers—real or perceived—that may hinder you in making positive lifestyle choices.

Identify your roadblocks

Any major lifestyle change is going to come with some roadblocks, which is completely natural. The most important thing is to not view these roadblocks as a reason to give up, because they're actually exactly what you need to achieve success. Rather than viewing roadblocks as a reason you can't succeed, embrace them as a challenge. With success comes amazing benefits.

> **Information is power.** Every time you hit a roadblock, you have more information on why you may not have succeeded in the past and an idea of what you need to do to succeed in the future.

> **Be honest with yourself**. There's no shame in admitting what you're finding hard. Your road to success is a personal one and needs to be tailored to your needs. For example, if you find it too hard to prepare a meal after getting home from work, this doesn't mean you can't eat an optimal diet. You just now know that one of your keys to success will be finding strategies to make this as easy as possible.

> **Share your journey.** One of the great strengths of the CHIP experience is that you are sharing it with a group of like-minded people, who are dealing with similar challenges. Talking about roadblocks is great, because you can come across some great tips that others have used to overcome these challenges. Share the tips you've found work for you for other roadblocks and make a positive difference in someone else's journey, too.

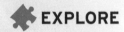 **EXPLORE**

Read *Learn More*, Chapter Fourteen

> What percentage of our health outcomes are influenced by our choices?

....

....

....

....

> What is the most powerful way to change the genetic "switch setting"?

....

....

....

> Do you know any identical twins? In what ways are they different, despite being genetically "identical"?

....

....

....

> How does our lifestyle affect future generations?

....

....

....

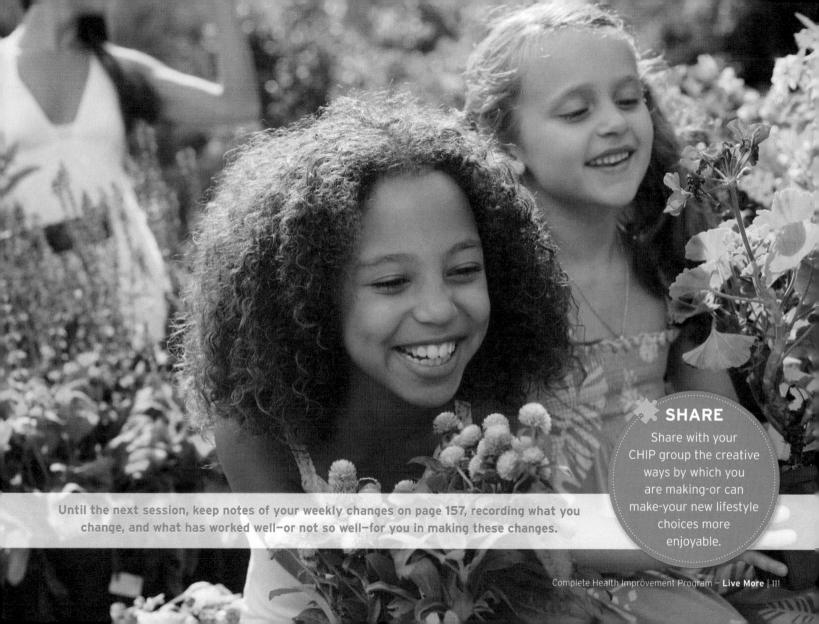

SHARE

Share with your CHIP group the creative ways by which you are making-or can make-your new lifestyle choices more enjoyable.

Until the next session, keep notes of your weekly changes on page 157, recording what you change, and what has worked well—or not so well—for you in making these changes.

Practising Forgiveness

🧩 DISCOVER

› What three things have you learned?

....

....

....

....

› In what different ways can anger be expressed?

....

....

....

....

"Unforgiveness is like carrying around a red-hot rock with the intention of throwing it at the person who caused you the hurt. But as you wait . . . the sizzling rock burns and scars your hand."

[Dr Dick Tibbits]

> What effects does anger have on the vascular system?

....

....

....

> How do we put the past in the past where it belongs?

....

....

....

> What are the benefits of forgiving?

....

....

....

> Who benefits most from forgiveness?

....

....

> If not about forgetting, what is the goal of forgiveness?

....

....

....

> What does it mean to reframe a past event?

....

....

....

› How can you reframe a past event?

....

....

....

› Dr Tibbits says that "Forgiveness is the one thing that changes everything!" Do you agree? Explain your answer.

....

....

....

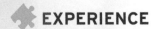 **EXPERIENCE**

› Write a letter to someone you wish to forgive in order to let go of a painful experience from your past. Use the page opposite to write this letter of forgiveness and experience the freedom to move on and put this experience behind you.

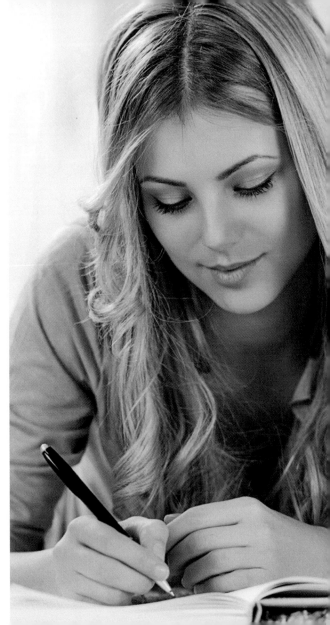

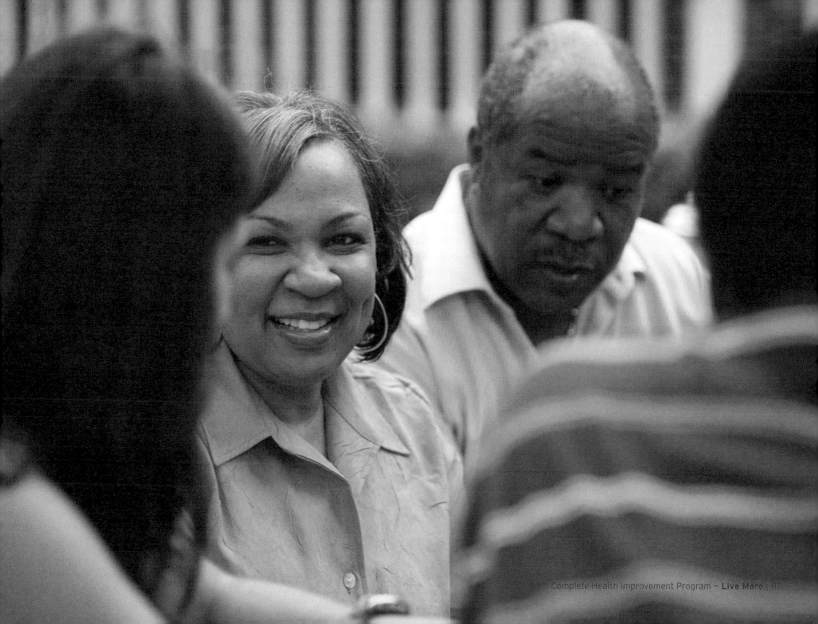

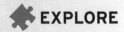 **EXPLORE**

Read *Learn More,* Chapter Thirteen

> What are the two options for dealing with anger? Can you think of other options?

....

....

....

....

> Complete the sentence: "Forgiveness is not . . ."

....

....

....

> Thinking about a specific case where you need to forgive, at what point are you in the Stages of Change diagram in relation to this specific case? What do you need to do to move to the next stage?

....

....

....

....

....

....

....

STAGES OF CHANGE *(relapse–can occur at any stage)*				
Pre-contemplation	**Contemplation**	**Preparation**	**Action**	**Maintenance/ Relapse**
Do you remember a time when you weren't concerned about your health or didn't see any need to change anything?	At some point, you began to consider the possibility that you needed to do something. Some people think about it for months, years or even their entire lives without progressing.	You began to prepare for the change–bought a pair of running shoes, researched gym memberships or began looking for healthy recipes.	Then you took action: perhaps you started walking during your lunch break. It was great! You felt good about yourself. You could feel your body toning up. You didn't get so puffed going up the hill.	But for how long were you able to maintain it? Were you derailed by a week of non-stop rain? The end-of-financial-year pressures in the office? A family crisis?

› In what areas do you need to forgive yourself?

....

....

....

Until the next session, keep notes of your weekly changes on page 157, recording what you change, and what has worked well–or not so well–for you in making these changes.

SHARE

Read your forgiveness letter to someone you trust, and if safe to do so, send it to the person concerned. Only do what you are comfortable with!

Re-engineering Your Environment

🧩 DISCOVER

› What three things have you learned?

....

....

....

....

› What can you do to make better choices at home?

....

....

....

....

Our modern environment supports obesity–it is "obesogenic."

› What can you do to make better choices at the grocery store?

....

....

....

....

....

› What can you do to make better choices at work?

....

....

....

....

› What can you do to make better choices when eating out?

....

....

....

....

....

› What can you do to make better choices when traveling?

....

....

....

....

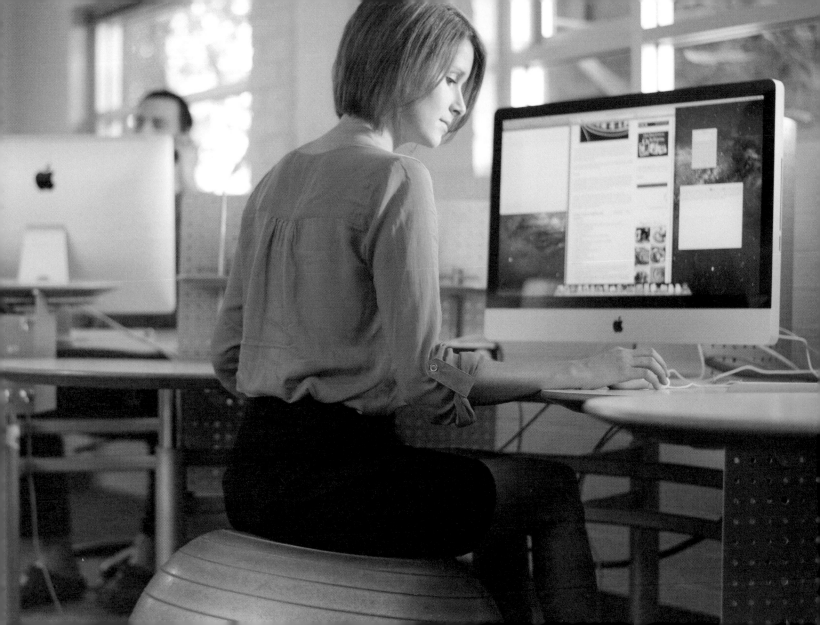

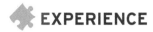 **EXPERIENCE**

Re-engineer your environment

Our changing environment has played a large role in the rise of obesity. In fact, many of us live in an "obesogenic" environment! Changes in our work, shopping, entertainment and recreation can all work against us without us even realizing it. One key to success when it comes to securing a healthier lifestyle in the long-term is to re-engineer our environment so it supports healthy behaviors.

Identify some things you can change about your physical surroundings that will force you to practise healthier habits.

› Look carefully at your work environment and find strategies to reduce sit time. For example, move your telephone to a place where you have to stand up when using it. Connect to a printer that requires you to walk to pick up your printing.

› Move the "sweets bowl" if you find it difficult to resist—or fill it with healthy items.

› Put a treadmill or exercise bike in front of the television at home.

› In your work and home environment, how can you reduce the amount of time that you spend looking at screens? What alternatives are there to screen time?

› Be selective about what aisles you allow yourself to walk down when you do your grocery shopping.

In all your interactions with your environment ask yourself: "How can I make healthy choices in this situation?"

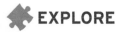 **EXPLORE**

Read *Learn More*, Chapter Fifteen

> What is the real cause of the
> obesity epidemic?

....

....

....

....

....

....

> In what ways is your social environment
> supporting or not supporting the healthy
> choices that you are making? What steps can
> you take to make it more supportive?

....

....

....

....

....

....

› In what ways can you adapt your physical surroundings to support the healthy choices that you are making?

....

....

....

....

....

....

Until the next session, keep notes of your weekly changes on page 159, recording what you change, and what has worked well—or not so well—for you in making these changes.

SHARE
With a colleague or family member, re-engineer something in your joint environment.

Session Sixteen

Stress-relieving Strategies

✦ DISCOVER

› What three things have you learned?

....

....

....

....

....

....

....

› Thinking of a time when you have experienced the "stress response", describe the symptoms that you felt.

....

....

....

....

› List some sources of stress in your life.

....

....

....

....

› What effects can ongoing stress have on your health?

....

....

....

....

› Were you surprised to learn that researchers from Ohio State University found that wounds took 30 per cent longer to heal following an argument than following a pleasant interaction with a partner? Why?

....

....

....

....

› What steps can you take to limit your stress?

....

....

....

....

› What did you experience during the "relaxation response" exercise?

....

....

....

....

....

Experience the relaxation response at <www.vimeo.com/chiphealth>.

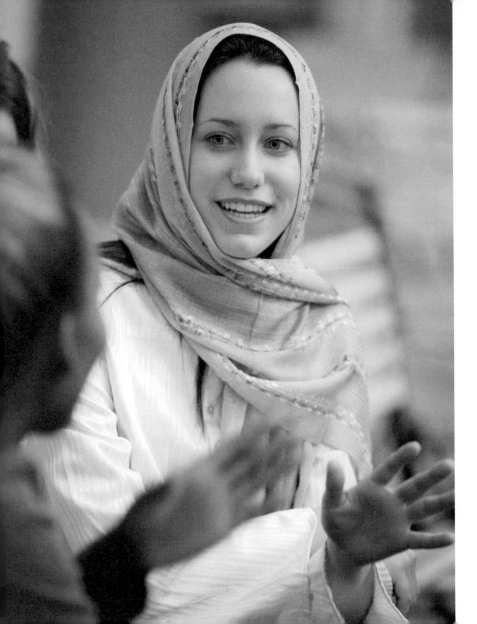

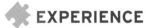 **EXPERIENCE**

Find a strategy that helps you stress less:

We have just learned that "Stress can wreak havoc with your metabolism, raise your blood pressure, burst your white blood cells, make you flatulent, ruin your sex life, and if that's not enough, possibly damage your brain." Unless we implement positive strategies toward dealing with stress it can overwhelm us.

> Make a list of the issues causing you stress today. Divide the list into two columns; those you have control over and those you haven't. Select one item that you do have control over and make a plan to deal with that issue within the next 24 hours.

> Find someone you trust, and talk to them about your stress.

> Develop strategies for incorporating more exercise into your daily routine.

> Practise the "relaxation response" twice today

> Find your "happy place"–a place where you feel relaxed and at peace. Plan to spend some time there in the next few days.

YOUR STRESS

YOUR CONTROL

	Yes	No
Example: Struggle to maintain balance between work life and home life.	✓	☐
	☐	☐
	☐	☐
	☐	☐
	☐	☐
	☐	☐
	☐	☐
	☐	☐
	☐	☐
	☐	☐
	☐	☐

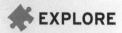 **EXPLORE**

Read *Learn More*, Chapter Sixteen

> In what ways does how you feel affect your health?

....

....

....

> In what ways does exercise help to relieve stress?

....

....

....

> Can you relate to Mark Twain's comment "I have known a great many troubles, but most of them have never happened."?

....

....

> How does talking to someone else about stress help to reduce the stress?

....

....

....

....

....

> Who can you share with openly and honestly about the things that cause you stress and how it affects you?

....

....

....

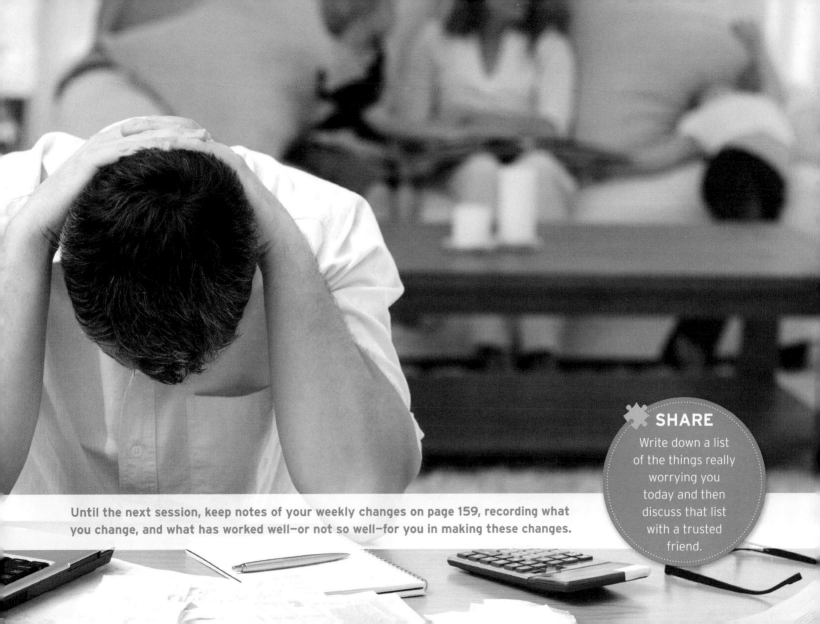

Until the next session, keep notes of your weekly changes on page 159, recording what you change, and what has worked well—or not so well—for you in making these changes.

SHARE

Write down a list of the things really worrying you today and then discuss that list with a trusted friend.

Session Seventeen

Fix How You Feel

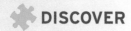 **DISCOVER**

› What three things have you learned?

....

....

....

....

....

....

....

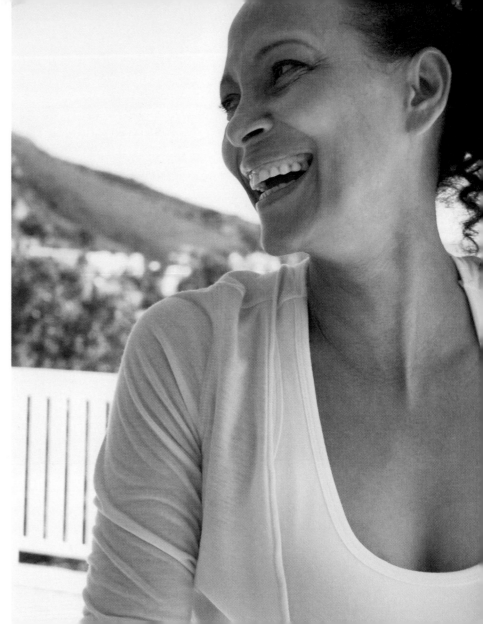

> Did you find it interesting to learn that people who lacked exposure to nature were more prone to anxiety and depression? Explain your answer.

....

....

....

....

....

> What two elements of the natural world are described as being the most important?

....

....

....

....

> The five tips that can fix how you feel are: eat highly nutritious foods; move dynamically; go natural; rest well; and look up. Which two of these five areas do you need to invest additional time in?

....

....

....

....

> How does the law that "you reap what you sow" apply to your emotions?

....

....

....

....

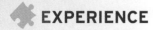 **EXPERIENCE**

> Write a gratitude letter to someone who's had a significant impact on your life. Use the page opposite to write this letter.

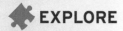 **EXPLORE**

Read *Learn More*, **Chapter Seventeen**

> What do you think are the key factors that determine your quality of life?

....

....

....

....

....

> What steps can you take to improve the quality of your sleep?

....

....

....

....

....

> This chapter suggests a "Sabbath" principle of taking one day a week off. How can you begin to incorporate this principle into your lifestyle?

....

....

....

> What in life are you truly thankful for?

....

....

....

....

> What in life are you truly excited about?

....

....

....

....

> What can you do to make someone else feel good?

....

....

....

SHARE

Tell someone something that you are truly thankful for and excited about.

Until the next session, keep notes of your weekly changes on page 159, recording what you change, and what has worked well—or not so well—for you in making these changes.

Session Eighteen

From Surviving to Thriving

✦ DISCOVER

> What three things have you learned?

> In what way did Dr Michael Norton (Harvard Business School) find that money could buy happiness? Was the amount of money involved significant?

While happiness is a worthy pursuit, it takes more than just smiles and giggles to thrive in life.

> List the five domains that constitute a life that truly flourishes.

P ....

E ....

A ....

R ....

M ....

> In what ways do you have meaning in your life? What gives you meaning in life?

....

....

....

....

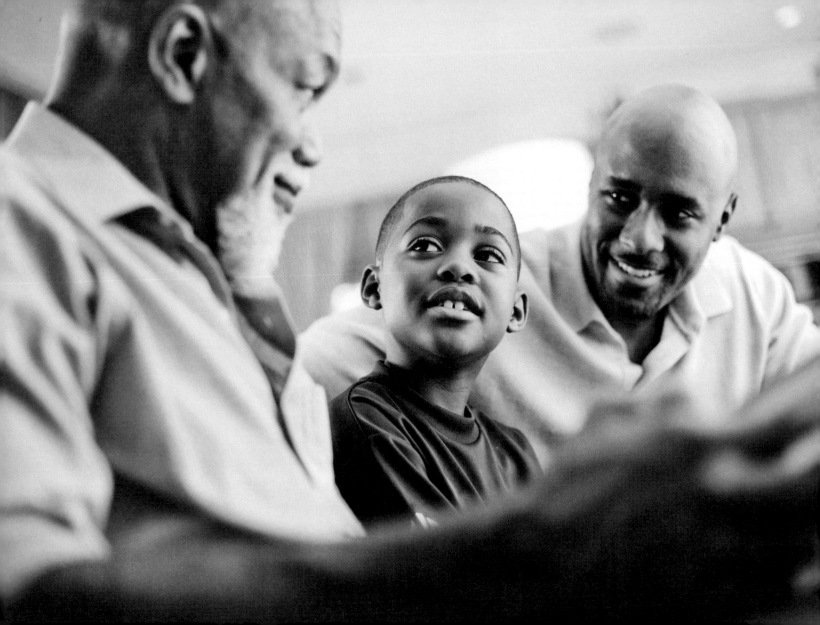

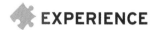 **EXPERIENCE**

Pass it on

In order to live a life that flourishes, there are five components summarized in the acronym PEARM: Positive Emotion, Engagement, Achievement, Relationships and Meaning. The deepest level of flourishing comes through meaning, which Dr Seligman defines as "belonging to and serving something that you believe is bigger than the self." It is about making a real difference in someone else's life. Today's prescription is for you to choose to make a difference in the lives of those around you.

> Undertake a random act of kindness—do something to help a total stranger.

> Utilize your signature strength to help someone else.

> Take the time to get to know the names of five children or teenagers in your community—research shows that it does them wonders.

> Take note of when someone you're working with does something well and affirm them for it.

> Buy some flowers or other gift to give to someone you appreciate.

> Tell someone close to you about what you have discovered in the CHIP program and the difference it has made to you.

> Volunteer to help out in the next CHIP program.

Only when we recognize that our strengths and skills are for service, not status, do we truly come alive.

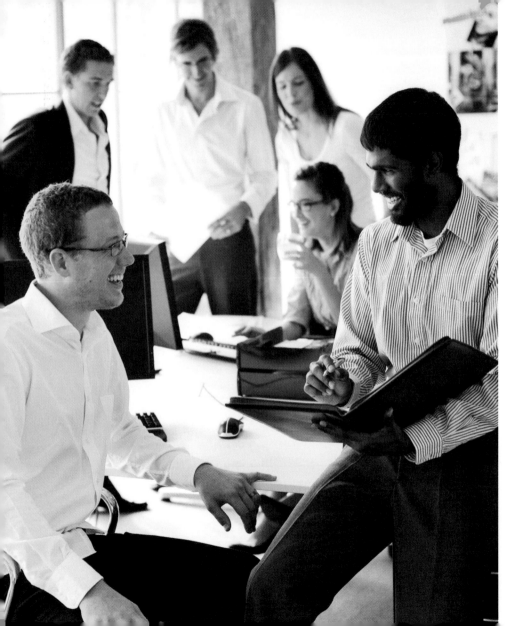

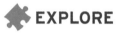 **EXPLORE**

Read *Learn More*, Chapter Eighteen

> What are the limitations of positive emotions?

....

....

....

....

> Describe a situation where you have felt totally engaged in what you do.

....

....

....

....

....

> List three significant things you have achieved.

....

....

....

....

> What relationships do you have that contribute to other people's lives?

....

....

....

....

> Dr Martin Seligman defines meaning as a feeling of "belonging to and serving something that you believe is bigger than the self." In what way is this true in your life?

....

....

....

....

....

....

SHARE
Perform a random act of kindness (for a stranger or someone you care about).

Keep notes of your weekly changes on page 160, recording what you change, and what has worked well—or not so well—for you in making these changes.

Recording Your CHIP Journey

Throughout *Live More*, you'll be invited to record a number of things about your CHIP journey, including test results, things that have worked well for you and challenges you've faced. This section of *Live More* is devoted to just that, so when you want to look back on your progress or jog your memory on a strategy that's worked well for you, you can turn to one simple section. So if you're looking for tools that will help you keep track of your journey to health, here they are.

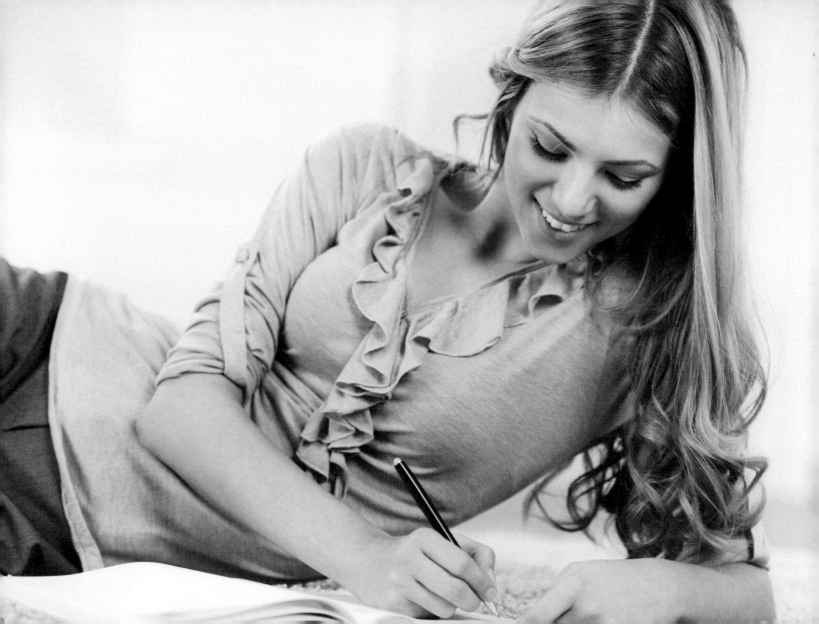

Personal Goal and Action Plan

RECORD YOUR RESULTS

	BEFORE		PROGRESS 1		PROGRESS 2	
	Date	Result	Date	Result	Date	Result
Weight						
Height						
Waist Measurement						
Blood Pressure (mmHg)						
Blood Glucose						
Total Cholesterol						
LDL Cholesterol						
Triglycerides						
HDL Cholesterol						

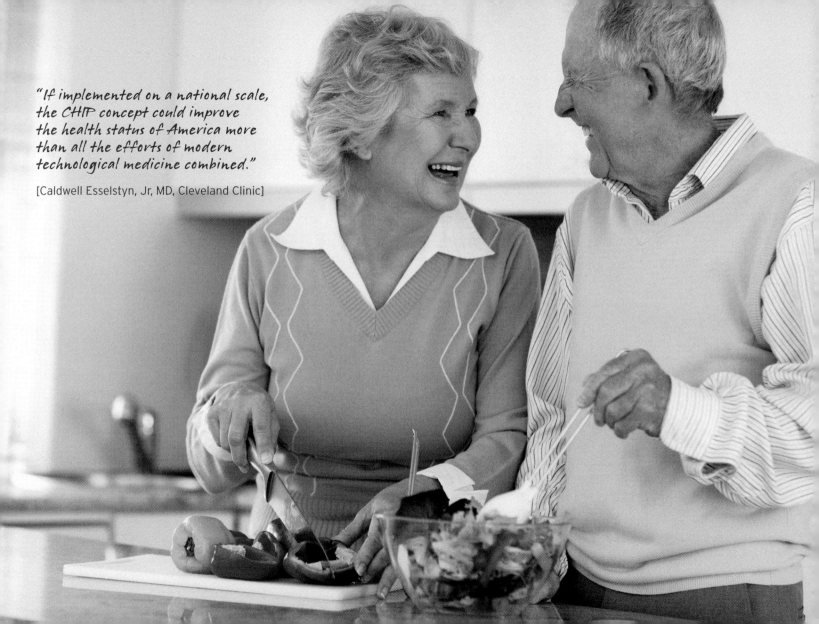

"If implemented on a national scale, the CHIP concept could improve the health status of America more than all the efforts of modern technological medicine combined."

[Caldwell Esselstyn, Jr, MD, Cleveland Clinic]

Your Daily Physical Activity Target

Your goal is to achieve 10,000 steps a day and the most simple way to know when you have achieved this target is by wearing your pedometer and placing one foot in front of the other until "10,000" appears on the screen (but don't feel you have to stop there).

Alternatively, if you find your pedometer has a habit of forgetting to attach itself to your person, or you like performing physical activities that pedometers aren't good at counting (for example, swimming, cycling or resistance exercises), here is another way to achieve your 10,000 target.

The first 5000 steps are awarded for simply getting out of bed and moving somewhat throughout the course of the day. So far so good!—but still make an effort not to sit for too long uninterrupted. The remaining 5000 steps you have to earn. You can achieve them by engaging in moderate-intensity physical activity—that which requires about a 3 or 4 out of 10 in effort (you can talk but not sing). For every 10 minutes of moderate-intensity exercise, you get 1000 steps and, of course, you don't have to do the 10-minute chunks all in the one hit. If you enjoy more vigorous-intensity exercise—say a 5 or more out of 10 in effort in which you can't hold a conversation without catching a breath—you get credited with 1000 steps for every 5 minutes. Consider resistance exercises as "moderate-intensity" (10 minutes = 1000 steps). Even though you might put in a big effort while performing the exercise, there is usually quite a bit of rest between sets. Note that it is also OK to mix and match moderate-intensity, vigorous-intensity and resistance exercises to achieve your target.

RECAP: Your target is 10,000 steps or equivalent per day.

Record your daily activity level in the tables provided on the following pages by either:

> Recording the number of steps counted by your pedometer.

OR

> Crediting yourself with 5000 steps for your general daily movements and then achieving 1000 steps for every 10 minutes of moderate-intensity exercise or 5 minutes of vigorous-intensity exercise.

Use this activity diary to note down all the activity you've incorporated into your month

	WEEK 1 Date:_____		WEEK 2 Date:_____		WEEK 3 Date:_____		WEEK 4 Date:_____	
	Activity	Count	Activity	Count	Activity	Count	Activity	Count
Sunday	Got off bus one stop earlier and walk the rest	20 mins						
	Lunchtime brisk walk	10 mins						
	Pedometer daily total	8452						
Monday								
Tuesday								
Wednesday								
Thursday								
Friday								
Saturday								

Use this activity diary to note down all the activity you've incorporated into your month

	WEEK 1 Date:_____		WEEK 2 Date:_____		WEEK 3 Date:_____		WEEK 4 Date:_____	
	Activity	Count	Activity	Count	Activity	Count	Activity	Count
Sunday								
Monday								
Tuesday								
Wednesday								
Thursday								
Friday								
Saturday								

Use this activity diary to note down all the activity you've incorporated into your month

	WEEK 1 Date:_____		WEEK 2 Date:_____		WEEK 3 Date:_____		WEEK 4 Date:_____	
	Activity	Count	Activity	Count	Activity	Count	Activity	Count
Sunday								
Monday								
Tuesday								
Wednesday								
Thursday								
Friday								
Saturday								

Note Your Weekly Changes

Record what you change, and what has worked well—or not so well—for you in making these changes.

SESSION 1

....

....

....

....

SESSION 2

....

....

....

....

SESSION 3

SESSION 4

SESSION 5

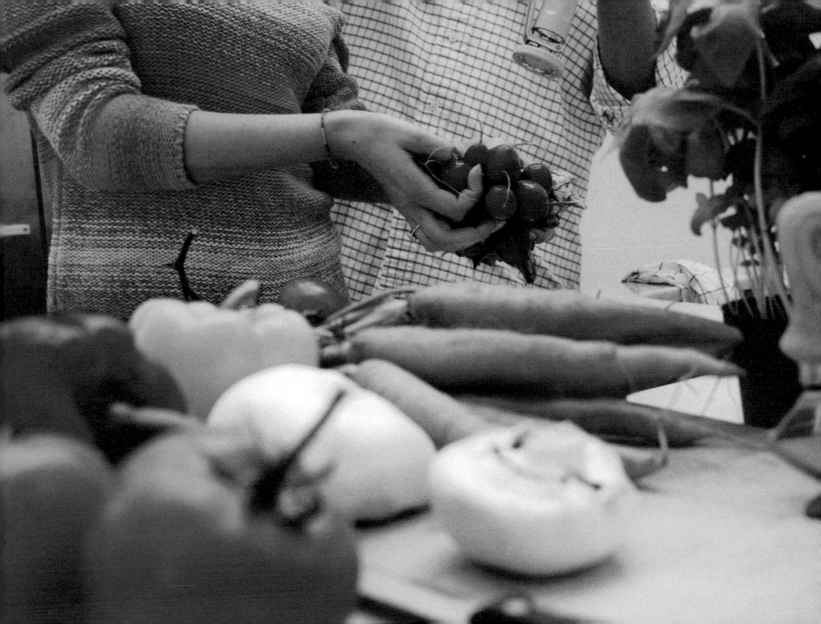

SESSION 6

SESSION 7

SESSION 8

SESSION 9

....

....

....

SESSION 10

....

....

....

SESSION 11

....

....

....

SESSION 12

SESSION 13

SESSION 14

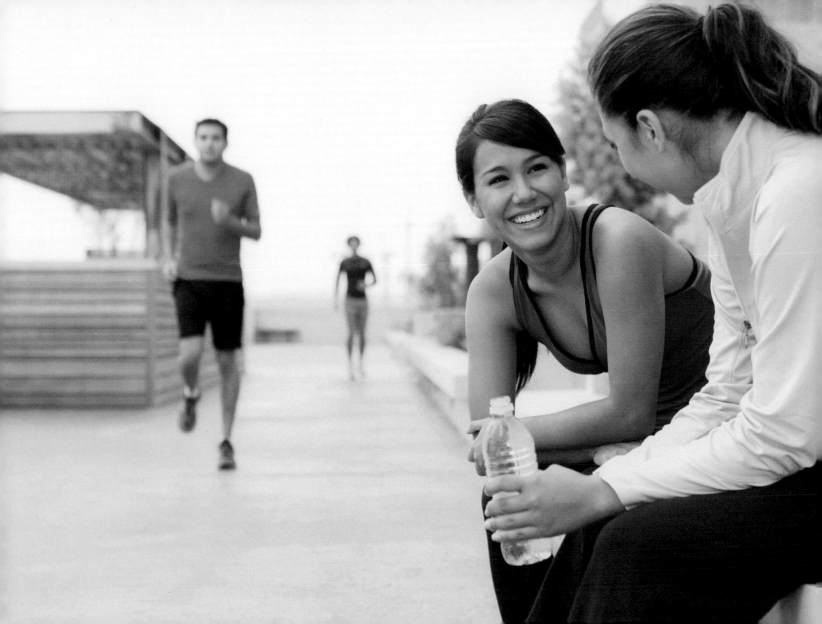

SESSION 15

....

....

....

SESSION 16

....

....

....

SESSION 17

....

....

....

NOTES

[Whole grains (fiber)] - Polenta, (Oats), (Quinoa), (Ragi), Bulgar, Buckwheat, Farro, Millet, (Barley), Brown Rice, Teff, (Edamame noodles), Sprouted bread (Trader Joe's)

(PROTEIN): Lentils, Beans, Tofu

Good Snack options] - Fruits, vegetables, whole grain nuts, hummus, plant-based proteins,
Almonds, Pecans, Walnuts